MW00736934

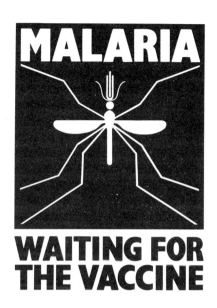

MALARIA

WAITING FOR THE VACCINE

London School of Hygiene and Tropical Medicine
First Annual Public Health Forum

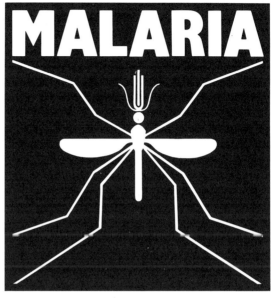

MALARIA

WAITING FOR THE VACCINE

Edited by

G.A.T. Targett

*London School of Hygiene
and Tropical Medicine*

JOHN WILEY & SONS

Chichester · New York · Brisbane · Toronto · Singapore

Copyright © 1991 by John Wiley & Sons Ltd
Baffins Lane, Chichester
West Sussex PO19 1UD, England

All rights reserved.

No part of this book may be reproduced by any means,
or transmitted, or translated into a machine language
without the written permission of the publisher.

Other Wiley Editorial Offices

John Wiley & Sons, Inc., 605 Third Avenue,
New York, NY 10158-0012, USA

Jacaranda Wiley Ltd, G.P.O. Box 859, Brisbane,
Queensland 4001, Australia

John Wiley & Sons (Canada) Ltd, 22 Worcester Road,
Rexdale, Ontario M9W 1L1, Canada

John Wiley & Sons (SEA) Pte Ltd, 37 Jalan Pemimpin 05-04,
Block B, Union Industrial Building, Singapore 2057

Library of Congress Cataloging-in-Publication Data

London School of Hygiene and Tropical Medicine. Public Health Forum
(1st : 1991 : London, England)
    Malaria, waiting for the vaccine / London School of Hygiene and
Tropical Medicine First Annual Public Health Forum ; edited by G.
Targett.
        p.   cm.
    Forum held April 1991 in London.
    Includes bibliographical references.
    ISBN 0 471 93100 4
    1. Malaria—Preventive inoculation—Congresses.   I. Targett, G.
II. Title.
    [DNLM: 1. Malaria—drug therapy—congresses.   2. Malaria—
immunology—congresses.   3. Malaria—prevention & control—
congresses.   4. Vaccines—congresses.   WC 750 L8475m]
RA644.M2L65   1991
614.5'32—dc20
DNLM/DLC
for Library of Congress   91-40008
                                                               CIP

British Library Cataloguing-in-Publication Data

A catalogue record for this book is
available from the British Library

ISBN 0 471 93100 4

Typeset in 10/12pt Times by APS, Salisbury, Wilts
Printed and bound in Great Britain by Biddles Ltd, Guildford and King's Lynn

Contents

Contributors

Alberto Alzate Facultad de Salud, Universidad del Valle, Apartado Aereo 25360, Cali, Colombia

Lu Bao Lin Institute of Microbiology and Epidemiology, 27 Taiping Road, Beijing 100850, People's Republic of China

Anders Björkman Department of Infectious Diseases, Karolinska Institute, Roslagstull Hospital, S-114 89 Stockholm, Sweden

Bernard J. Brabin Department of Tropical Paediatrics, Liverpool School of Tropical Medicine, Pembroke Place, Liverpool L3 5QA, UK

David J. Bradley Department of Epidemiology and Population Sciences, London School of Hygiene and Tropical Medicine, Keppel Street, London WC1E 7HT, UK

Pierre Carnevale Antenne Orstom aupres de l'OCEAC, BP 288, Yaounde, Cameroun

Christopher F. Curtis Department of Medical Parasitology, London School of Hygiene and Tropical Medicine, Keppel Street, London WC1E 7HT, UK

Susan D. F. Foster Department of Public Health and Policy, London School of Hygiene and Tropical Medicine, Keppel Street, London, WC1E 7HT, UK

Brian M. Greenwood Medical Research Laboratories, Fajara, Banjul, The Gambia

Richard J. Hayes Department of Epidemiology and Population Sciences, London School of Hygiene and Tropical Medicine, Keppel Street, London, WC1E 7HT, UK

Ralph H. Henderson Assistant Director-General, World Health Organization, 1211 Geneva 27, Switzerland

Somkid Kaewsonthi The Centre for Health Economics, Faculty of Economics, Chulalongkorn University, Bangkok, Thailand

Penelope J. Key   Senior Health and Population Advisor, Overseas Development Administration, Victoria Street, London SW1E 5JL, UK

Fenella Kirkham   Institute of Child Health, Guilford Street, London WC1, UK

Bernard H. Liese   Director, Health Services Department, World Bank, 1818 H Street NW, Washington, DC 20433, USA

Kevin Marsh   Kenya Medical Research Institute, PO Box 428, Kilifi, Kenya

Kamini N. Mendis   Department of Parasitology, Faculty of Medicine, University of Colombo, Kynsey Road, Colombo 8, Sri Lanka

Louis H. Miller   Malaria Section, Laboratory of Parasitic Diseases, National Institute of Allergy and Infectious Diseases, National Institutes of Health, Bethesda, MD 20892, USA

Anne Mills   Department of Public Health and Policy, London School of Hygiene and Tropical Medicine, Keppel Street, London WC1E 7HT, UK

Louis Molineaux   Operational Research, Division of Control of Tropical Diseases, World Health Organization, 1211 Geneva 27, Switzerland

Charles R.J.C. Newton   Nuffield Department of Paediatrics, John Radcliffe Hospital, Headington, Oxford OX9 3DU, UK

Phuc Nguyen-Dinh   Malaria Branch, Division of Parasitic Diseases, Centers for Disease Control, Atlanta, GA 30333, USA

John H.L. Playfair   Department of Immunology, University College and Middlesex Hospital Medical School, Arthur Stanley House, Tottenham Street, London W1P 9PG, UK

Vinod P. Sharma   Malaria Research Centre, 22 Sham Nath Marg, Delhi 110054, India

Peter G. Smith   Department of Epidemiology and Population Sciences, London School of Hygiene and Tropical Medicine, Keppel Street, London, WC1E 7HT, UK

Marcel Tanner   Department of Public Health and Epidemiology, Swiss Tropical Institute, Socinstrasse 57, CH-4002 Basel, Switzerland

Awash Teklehaimanot   Malaria Unit, World Health Organization, CTD/MAL, 1211 Geneva 27, Switzerland

J. Ben Were   Clinical Research Centre, Kemri, Nairobi

Nicholas J. White   Wellcome–Mahidol–Oxford University Tropical Medicine Research Programme, Faculty of Tropical Medicine, Mahidol University, Rajvithi Road, Bangkok 10400, Thailand

Peter A. Winstanley   Nuffield Department of Clinical Medicine, John Radcliffe Hospital, Headington, Oxford OX9 3DU, UK

Foreword

Figures quoted for the number of people in the world who are exposed to, contract, or die from malaria each year are inevitably only estimates, but this in no way lessens the reality of the disease. It has such a dominant and debilitating effect on huge populations, with fatalities (one million or more per annum) occurring most commonly in the children of the endemic regions.

The situation has been worsening in recent years with the seemingly inexorable spread of resistance to drugs shown by the parasite and to insecticides by the mosquito. Clearly much effort is being directed towards the development of new and effective means of combating both parasite and mosquito but, in the meantime, control must be attempted by use of combinations of methods most appropriate to each situation.

The First Annual Public Health Forum of the London School of Hygiene and Tropical Medicine brought together 200 experts from 54 countries. They represented every discipline concerned with the control of malaria, and provided invaluable advice on how best to cope at the national level, the community level, and the level of the individual sick child or adult. They also provided an informed view of expectations for the future. This book contains the considered opinions of selected experts and, importantly, a synthesis of the detailed discussions that took place on each dimension of the problem.

The ODA is delighted to be the major sponsor of the Forum and of this book. I hope it will be widely circulated and used as a guide by those who have to define the policies to be adopted in order to contain what is now a global problem that knows no boundaries.

The Rt Hon Lynda Chalker MP
Minister for Overseas Development, UK

Preface

This book is the product of the First Annual Public Health Forum of the London School of Hygiene and Tropical Medicine. The series was conceived to address each year a major issue in public health medicine that reflects the national and international role of the School in the subject. The choice of malaria as the subject for the first forum, and in particular the theme selected, was serendipitous given the subsequent international proposal that there should be a meeting of Health Ministers devoted specifically to malaria in 1992. The title, Malaria—Waiting for the Vaccine, was chosen to indicate that the debate would be on what to do now and in the near future, utilizing the resources currently available. It was recognized that the vaccines on which hopes are pinned are for the future and that there is an urgent need to ensure meanwhile that all other means of control are used to best effect. The School has expertise in malaria which is wide ranging, embracing laboratory sciences in immunology and chemotherapy on the one hand, through epidemiology and vector control, to the management and economics of health care programmes. This allowed us to construct a forum where experts from these many different disciplines could together address the issues with which each has to grapple, but this time in a multidisciplinary way and introducing we hoped some fresh ideas. We wanted everyone's thinking to be broadened. This objective was behind the establishment of workshops based on the same themes as the keynote addresses, the reports and recommendations from which are included here.

There is deliberately no index because the detail included, though considerable, is important mainly in the context of the policy being developed or recommended; whether for chemoprophylaxis, drug supply or future vaccine trials.

We owe a great debt of gratitude to the main sponsor of the meeting and the publication, the Overseas Development Administration of the British Foreign and Commonwealth Office. Their support also made it possible for delegates from some of the fifty-four countries represented at the meeting to attend. We are most grateful too for the generous support given by the World Health Organization, and by the World Bank and the Swiss Tropical Institute.

The organization of the forum within the School was a team effort and many colleagues deserve credit for its success. However, Barbara Judge and Andrea Bonsey had the pivotal roles and very special thanks go to them. The preparation of the book and its rapid publication were due in part to the authors allowing a considerable amount of editorial direction, but especially to Carolyn Brown and David FitzSimons of the Bureau of Hygiene and Tropical Diseases who took a large share of the early editorial work and later proof reading.

Richard Feachem
Dean
Geoffrey Targett
Conference Chairman and Editor

Introduction

MALARIA: CHALLENGES FOR THE 1990s

Penelope J. Key

Overseas Development Administration Senior Health and Population Adviser

I should first like to join my colleagues from the World Health Organization and the World Bank in congratulating the Dean and staff of the School on the occasion of the first Annual Public Health Forum — the first of a new series of important scientific meetings — to present and debate major public health issues pertinent to our times. I also congratulate the Dean for the vision and understanding which led him to choose malaria, one of the most serious of all health problems faced by people of the developing world. We are all only too well aware that in some parts of the world the malaria situation is getting worse rather than better: that malaria is responsible for high child death rates, for reduced economic production and for rendering considerable areas of land (hard-pressed in these times of rapidly growing population numbers) inaccessible to humans.

The ODA provided financial and representational support to the Forum. This demonstrated not only a recognition of the importance of the problem, but also an optimism and faith in all of the experts taking part who represented many specialist fields in — and related to — malaria: epidemiology, biology, economics, health policy, entomology and social science. We gathered to prove that it is not 'beyond the wit of the human mind' to solve this problem, caused by so small a parasite, working in efficient and close relationship with its complex vector mosquito.

I should like to reflect on my own personal involvement with this parasite and the disease and death resulting from its invasion of the human body. So little has changed since my first encounters with malaria nearly 30 years ago. Although it is worth mentioning that in the very early 1960s, when I was a medical student in London, I do not remember ever actually seeing a patient with malaria. In those days, travelling outside these islands for the majority of British people was unusual and travelling into malarious areas was for the adventurous few. How different the situation is now, with malaria being high on the differential diagnosis list for fever cases presenting in this country, and living close to an international airport here being a risk factor for contracting the disease.

I was one of those who went to practise my acquired skills in tropical countries, initially Papua New Guinea, one of those small Pacific countries well-represented at the Forum, where malaria still takes its toll of human life, both in quality and quantity, as it did when I first went there. I have two vivid memories to share: my first the huge spleens in the majority of the small children and the effect this chronic *Plasmodium vivax* infection had on the quality of their young lives; the second, the not infrequent presentation at clinic or small hospital of young women in late stages of pregnancy with haemoglobin levels so low as to almost defy the possibility of still being alive, let alone having in all probability walked long distances to seek treatment.

In those days it was the fashion to give weekly prophylactic chloroquine to pregnant women at antenatal clinics — yes, there were antenatal clinics held then and they were held out in the villages, often under trees, and they were well attended.

The issue of the time was whether to give prophylactic chloroquine to young babies and children, realizing fully the greater risk of the disease they would face when they stopped taking it and weighing this up against the high mortality risk of the first attack during the first year or two of life. *As I travel around now, visiting malaria endemic areas in the Pacific, in India, in South America, I notice that the issues have not changed, the disease has not changed, the risks have not changed—only the drugs have changed a little and our understanding of the nature of the infection has advanced.*

Those were also the days of DDT spraying; in every village and in every house the marks of the spray teams and the results of their visits were to be seen and noted. At first they were so welcome: they were marvellous at getting rid of bedbugs and other unwelcome visitors such as cockroaches and headlice, but the effect on domestic animals soon began to be noted, as cats and dogs suffered and died following the spray man's visits and teams were less careful about the disruption and general mess they caused. The issue of the day in the villages became how to evade the teams and how to avoid having your house sprayed.

In the early 1970s I went to another warm country where malaria was but one of a variety of risks. That country is Cambodia, represented at the Forum by two leading national scientists. Those were the days when we first started seeing *Plasmodium falciparum* cases not responding to the usual treatment regimes — the emerging problem of the parasite's ability to adapt and survive — and the new wonder drug Fansidar, later proved not to be the answer to everyone's prayers. The situation faced in this small, very poor South-East Asian country today probably demonstrates the worst scenario in the world, with side by side the resistant parasite, the resistant mosquito vector, and a group of people seriously debilitated by long years of insufficient and low-quality food supplies. But what are the solutions in that country or in any other similar country, where basic health infrastructure is largely deficient, where money is so scarce and what there is does not find its way into health service provision?

What can we as scientists offer and what can government organizations such as ODA do to help?

The main objective of the British Aid Programme is to improve the well-being of the poorest. ODA attempts to help partner governments establish conditions under which such improvements can be achieved — and sustained.

Within individual countries there are many competing demands on national budgets. The real value of health sector budgets is unlikely to increase substantially in the foreseeable future. Yet their growing numbers of people continue to face severe health problems and demand a range of services. We recognize that in the present economic circumstances many developing countries cannot sustain the level of health care that their people need, that legislators demand and, sometimes, that donor agencies encourage them to adopt.

ODA's health policy is to strengthen health systems and capacities so that they better support primary health care (PHC) in developing countries. The actual implementation of PHC has proved problematic. Much is demanded of PHC, and PHC workers, who have been faithfully recruited by many governments, are now being asked to provide a huge range of services, often without appropriate training or sufficient resources. Progress with development and implementation of PHC is being seriously hampered by one underlying problem — lack of money. We health professionals cannot ignore the severe economic crisis facing the majority of developing countries, their debt burden and the severe adjustment measures which they have had to adopt and which have affected so deeply what can and cannot be achieved. In this scenario, ODA, along with other donor organizations, has learned the bitter lesson of providing money for health sector developments which governments cannot possibly sustain after the external aid ends.

Where does malaria fit into this depressing scene? Perhaps most strikingly in our striving to sustain vertical national malaria control programmes, previously so effective. Many of us have experience of aid-financed supplies of insecticides, vehicles and spraying equipment lying in warehouses unused because governments have not been able to pay salaries for spray teams or provide fuel for vehicles to implement the programmes in the field.

As we consider the scientific solutions, we must take a responsible look at the context in which they are to be delivered and the realities faced by national governments as they go about the very difficult task of reforming their health sectors to take account of resource constraints. Health sector policies, including malaria control policies, must be realistic and must make the best use of the people, the land and the money at their disposal. Many countries will be unable to afford all the developments we have come to know as primary health care. They will have to assign priorities between specific interventions according to their effectiveness. We can help governments to examine more effective uses for their existing health investments; to look at improved financing and management procedures; to switch funds from curative to preventive services; to analyse critically the numbers and types of health personnel needed to deliver services — all alternatives to more staff and higher budgets. We must not ask for innovations and changes that do not fit in with a country's carefully developed systems and structures.

ODA expects to do more of this. To help us, we are encouraging British institutions to strengthen their capacity in these subjects: planning, management, financing and evaluation. We are working with both the London School of Hygiene and Tropical Medicine and the Liverpool School of Tropical Medicine on a number of major programmes to tackle the health and population problems of fundamental concern to developing countries. One of these at the London School deals with the epidemiology and control of major tropical parasitic infections, including malaria. The challenge for these programmes, as to all of us, is to develop solutions to the identified problem which meet each individual community's health needs and aspirations, and which, at the same time, are also effective, affordable and sustainable.

As we suggest malaria-specific activities we must ask ourselves:

- Are the necessary recurrent funds likely to be available in the foreseeable future? If not, what is an alternative?
- Are there the people, the institutions and the management systems available to implement the strategies successfully?

Health professionals have to accept the introduction of cost consciousness in health systems and understand that value for money and control of expenditure are equally valid contributors to health development as quality, coverage and impact of care. This is a major consideration for ODA in the support we will give to health and population developments in the 1990s.

ODA reaffirms its support for the objectives set out here and will consider seriously the recommendations made for future policy and planning in malaria control. We have every intention of continuing that support by providing assistance to other preparatory meetings in different parts of the world, and to the global summit meeting in 1992.

MALARIA AND THE WORLD HEALTH ORGANIZATION

Ralph H. Henderson

Assistant Director-General, World Health Organization, Geneva, Switzerland

Malaria still remains among the three or four most devastating diseases occurring in the world today, and it is estimated that around 100 million clinical cases may occur every year in tropical Africa alone, where changes in the epidemiological situation have resulted in the last few years in an increased frequency of the disease, often of epidemic proportions, in areas such as Ethiopia, Madagascar, Rwanda and northern Sudan. In other parts of the world, while malaria remains under control in most developed and stable areas, the situation is dramatically deteriorating in all frontier areas of economic development, i.e. in areas where the exploitation of natural resources or illegal trade occurs, in jungle areas or areas burdened with problems of civil war and other conflicts, and where mass movements of refugees exist. Increasing drug resistance, decreasing efficacy of vector control efforts, weak health infrastructure and the progressive decay of outmoded managerial structures also affect control of this disease.

These conditions led both the WHO Executive Board and the World Health Assembly in 1989 to pass resolutions affirming that malaria control must remain a global priority essential for the achievement of health for all and the objectives of child survival programmes. Further, during the January 1990 session of the Executive Board, members considered the situation to be so serious they recommended that a global ministerial conference should be held. The objectives of this meeting, to be hosted by the Government of the Netherlands in October 1992, will be to focus the attention of endemic countries and donor agencies on the rapidly worsening malaria situation, to strengthen the commitment to malaria control among political and health leaders of member states and among donor agencies, and to improve and support a global plan of action for malaria control.

There are no simple solutions to the world's malaria problem and no single strategy for control will be applicable to all countries and all epidemiological situations. Experience has shown that, in most parts of the world, malaria is a disease which can be neither eradicated nor controlled by the 'campaign' approach in which a single package of interventions is implemented intensively for a limited period. Nevertheless, it is possible to identify strategic principles which are globally valid and fundamental to the operation of all control programmes. They can be formulated as four recommendations:

(1) Timely and adequate diagnosis and treatment of malarial disease should be provided as a basic right of all populations at risk of malaria. This, if correctly applied from the periphery to hospital level of the health services and targeted to populations at greatest risk of severe illness and death, will prevent most mortality.

(2) Vector control activities should be used selectively where they are cost effective and their achievements can be sustained. The decision on whether to apply vector control and the selection of tools to be used will depend on the local identification of epidemiological types.

(3) Early-warning systems should be developed which detect both the risk and existence of epidemics, complemented by systems which facilitate the rapid deployment of control interventions.

(4) Routine information systems should be developed which can provide timely data of relevance to monitor the local malaria situation and to permit the timely selection and application of control options as required.

The WHO is currently discussing and refining this approach to malaria control through a series of meetings prior to the 1992 ministerial conference. We believe the outcome of the Forum, *Malaria—Waiting for the Vaccine*, provides information which will help the WHO and, particularly, malaria endemic countries in developing practical solutions to the multiple facets of the problem which this disease presents.

With major emphasis of the strategy being placed on the easy access to diagnosis and treatment of the total population at risk, it will be necessary to strengthen and improve the capacity of health systems to manage common diseases, particularly fever, at the community level. This should be supported by effective referral systems for cases of severe malaria and treatment failures. These services can also provide an effective mechanism for the promotion of the use of individual protection methods, and form the basis for early-warning systems for epidemics and for detecting the evolution of parasite resistance to drugs. Information from the health services will also identify areas where more complex interventions for curbing transmission should be introduced. In most of Africa and the frontier areas of economic development where a health infrastructure is lacking or rudimentary, the application of this principle will first require building the necessary health infrastructure. Outside tropical Africa in countries where antimalarial programmes exist, the challenge will be to replan, reorient, retrain and redistribute existing resources where outmoded practices and infrastructures of previous eradication programmes continue to be used.

During the last decade there has been a renaissance in laboratory and clinical research on malaria. This is essential, since most of the available interventions are far from ideal, not only in their effectiveness but also in their suitability for incorporation into routine control activities. Unfortunately, there is often a polarization between control programmes and research institutes so that many research projects have little relevance to the needs of the local control programmes. In addition, control staff have generally not been trained in the specification of research questions relevant to the programmes' priorities and activities. Yet close collaboration between malaria research and malaria control is essential, for new tools and methodologies must be technically feasible for application in the field, and must be provided at a cost which is affordable by malaria-endemic countries. In the WHO, we are actively promoting this collaboration between researchers and controllers.

I would like to express the WHO's appreciation to the London School of Hygiene and Tropical Medicine for organizing this important meeting. I hope that our deliberations will provide a powerful springboard for our further work in preparing for the 1992 malaria ministerial conference.

MALARIA AND THE WORLD BANK

Bernhard H. Liese

Health Services Department, The World Bank

It may seem strange that the World Bank — whose principal function is to lend for development projects in order to strengthen the economies of borrowing countries — takes a keen interest in malaria.

The Bank does so because malaria is recognized as a major public health problem in so many of its borrower countries and because better health has always been viewed by the Bank as an important dimension of development. We are also involved because malaria can even be linked to specific development policies and actions — such as road building, new agricultural settlement and irrigation projects — and as such in itself constitutes an important aspect of development.

Bank lending for PHN projects has grown over the years, and in 1990 reached nearly a billion dollars in commitments. Lending for malaria control has likewise grown significantly, but has fluctuated. For example, in 1989 we approved US$120 million in loans for malaria control. This was the highest ever. In 1990 the lending was only about US$10 million. But more importantly the number of new projects with malaria control components has grown steadily.

The initial loans adopted the perspective that malaria was a development-related disease. Lending began in the early 1970s with support for distinct activities, as part of irrigation and other agricultural development projects. The amounts earmarked for malaria control were relatively small.

Later we began financing free-standing projects that supported malaria control activities on a larger scale. Still, these projects were basically in response to major agricultural development concerns. They were seen, in a way, as mitigating measures or complementary efforts to reduce the negative consequences of development on health.

More recently, in line with a general increase in interest in malaria and other tropical diseases among the major development institutions, we have taken a more pro-active approach. Accordingly, considerably larger sums have been approved. In addition, emergency situations — mostly malaria epidemics — have spurred efforts by the Bank to include support for malaria control in other loans and projects.

While our focus has naturally been on lending for malaria control activities — and here I include lending for local operational research — the Bank has also supported malaria research on an international scale. We have done this as a co-sponsor and through a substantial financial contribution to TDR (the Special

Programme for Training and Research in Tropical Diseases), a programme which we consider very important. We have also done some limited research in-house on topics such as tropical disease expenditures and more recently on the organization and management of successful tropical disease control programmes. Because even after five decades of malaria control half the world still lives at risk of malaria, we consider continued support for international research efforts as very important. We need new drugs and better control tools, and operational research to constantly adjust these control tools.

Let me return now to malaria and development, because this inescapable relationship seems to bring out the most important lessons we have learned from our own experience. In Brazil's Amazon, for example, we find rapid and disorderly migration of farmers, prospectors and entrepreneurs, increasing the vulnerability of native Indians — and an explosive growth of malaria. A combination of environmental, social, economic and even political factors have interacted to produce what has been labelled 'frontier malaria'. This malaria is by no means evenly distributed all over Amazonia — only 30 out of 450 municipalities account for 70% of all malaria. Furthermore, malaria is very localized in nature. In fact, resurgent malaria in Brazil today can be largely attributed to three major epidemiologically distinct areas: the famous gold-mining areas known as 'garimpos', the areas of new agricultural settlement and the rapidly expanding peripheral areas of Amazonian cities. We have been working closely with the Brazilian government and the international community to understand these locally diverse malaria situations, each of which has its own peculiar implications for control; and we have found what is true in Brazil holds for many other malarious countries as well.

Therefore, the first and foremost lesson we have learned is that there are a (limited) number of unique epidemiological situations — called 'patterns' — in most countries that require tailor-made control approaches. The earlier standardized single-measure strategies no longer suffice for effective malaria control. New more flexible combinations of control tools will be the key to future success.

Second, we have learned that the organization and management of disease control — that is, the institutional dimension — is as critical as technology development. Most importantly, the national ministries of health must be helped to develop the capacity to respond effectively to the newly identified patterns responsible for resurgent malaria. Governments must adopt deliberate policies to strengthen the malaria control organizations. This is especially important in Africa, where most of the world's malaria occurs, and which has not benefited from a long tradition of malaria control efforts.

We have learned some other important lessons as well: malaria had somehow disappeared for some years from the portfolio of international health priorities, but as the worldwide resurgence in malaria continues to grow, so does the threat to the well-being and productivity of millions of people. This is in stark contrast to the national health budgets, which are under increasing stress. It is therefore important that we help countries not only to intensify control but also to increase the effectiveness and efficiency of control efforts.

As for the future, the World Bank will continue to support projects and research activities for malaria control. But at the same time, we intend also to emphasize and advocate the very important task of putting malaria back on the map as a major priority in international public health, because malaria is not only a devastating tropical disease but is also a social condition closely associated with development.

Malaria—whence and whither?

David J. Bradley

London School of Hygiene and Tropical Medicine, UK

Introduction

While it is a great honour to provide the opening paper for the malaria conference and this book, it is also an intractable task to look briefly at the whole of malaria — past, present and future — and to try to meet the needs of such a diverse group as the conference participants and subsequent readers, who range from policy makers, with a breadth of wisdom and understanding but no special knowledge, to people who have devoted their whole lives to specific aspects of malariology. Yet there is some advantage to standing back and taking a bird's eye view, and more particularly to relating malaria control to more general concepts in public health. There is relevance in the comment of Lord Keynes that 'Every so-called practical politician is in reality the slave of some long-defunct ideology', and this extends beyond politicians to public health workers. This chapter looks for the underlying ideologies and concepts which, though we may be unaware of them, we continue to serve. I attempt to look at the wood, not the particular trees which will occupy others in this volume, and to focus on control strategy rather than parasitological research. In looking forwards, I shall suggest desirable trends and not point to new discoveries, for the very good reasons put forward by Sir Peter Medawar in his *Biological Retrospect*: that it is impossible to predict tomorrow's discoveries, except by making them, in which case they belong to today and not to the future.

The picture to be presented of the key issues will inevitably be oversimplified even though it will point towards greater complexity. It starts from just such a simplified dichotomous view of policies on how to control malaria. The theme for looking forwards will be one of continuity. Present action should be built upon the whole of past experience, and should not be simply a reaction to the immediately preceding period. To emphasize one issue in malaria control does not necessitate ignoring all others nor denigrating their role. At present there is rapid progress in malaria research, with the prospect of improvements in control, and great excitement. However, some of these improvements have been previously explored and it is unnecessary to reinvent the wheel and important not to ignore past work. The overall framework of malaria as an infection, disease and social problem is set out in Figure 1, to which the various discussions relate.

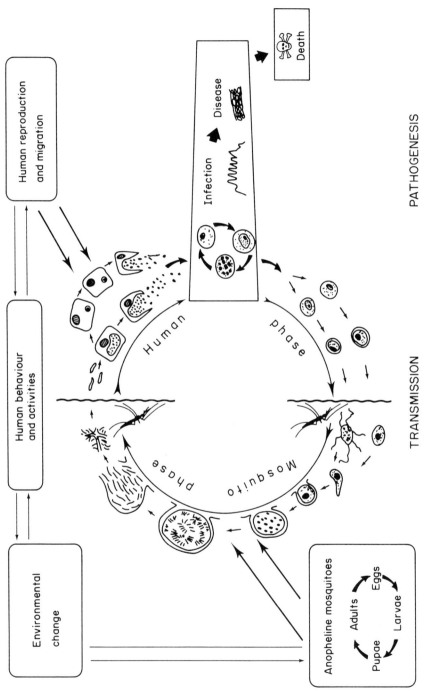

Figure 1 The transmission and pathogenesis of malaria: a diagram that includes social and environmental determinants

Table 1 Recent estimates of the numbers of people exposed to or suffering from malaria, expressed as an annual rate or period prevalence

Exposed	2 073 000 000
Infected	270 000 000
Ill	110 000 000
Died	1 000 000

But first it is necessary to consider the scale of the problem. All available figures are highly speculative, but a recent data set, of World Health Organization (WHO) origin, suggests the stark situation (Table 1). Enormous populations are involved. There is also a great difference between each successive pair of lines of the table. Moreover, the difference between the second and third lines would be much greater if both were expressed as point rather than period prevalences. These figures also point to the two key epidemiological questions about any infective disease: *regulation* and *variation*. These may be restated as: what is it that determines the level of malaria in the communities at risk; and why is it that many are infected, some are ill and far fewer (though still a great number) die? Which question dominates the scene depends on one's viewpoint — with variation fascinating the clinician and regulation of primary interest to the public health worker — and to some extent they are convergent questions, though regulation emphasizes similarities and variation stresses differences. These two aspects can well be epitomized by two of the great men of the past associated with the London School of Hygiene and Tropical Medicine and with malaria: Manson and Ross. As is well known, Manson can be taken to represent the clinical interest and approach while Ross's concern was for the community and public health (Figure 2). Such a stereotyping does not do justice to Manson's breadth of interest nor to the many-sided genius of Ross, but it helps to epitomize the two positions. These two different emphases perhaps mainly represent the partial vision of their followers and successors rather than the views of these two men, and both were highly relevant to research — Manson for his advocacy of the need for research, one of whose consequences was the founding of this School, and Ross for his personal research which both solved the key question of malaria transmission by mosquitoes and also laid the basis of epidemiological modelling.

Lessons from the past

The history of malaria was for many centuries (Table 2) about an increasing understanding of the circumstances under which it flourished, together with some preventive action, and a concurrent clinical understanding of the pattern of fever and association with splenomegaly that goes back to ancient China.

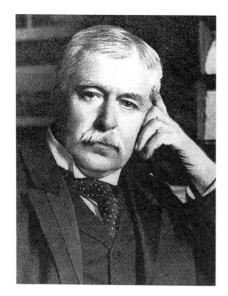

MANSON
Clinical
Person

PATHOGENESIS
Treatment
Patient

Risk approach

ROSS
Epidemiological
Community

TRANSMISSION
Control
Vector

Overall reduction

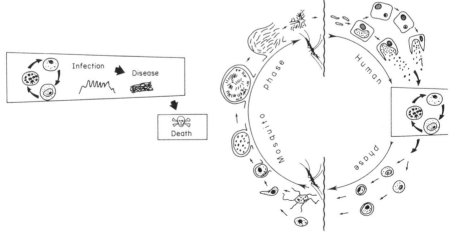

Figure 2   Two ways of looking at the problems of malaria, as epitomized by Sir Patrick
Manson and Sir Ronald Ross

Table 2 Some key events in the history of malaria and its control, with the time in years before the present at which each began to take place

5000	China: spleen and fever
2500	Hippocrates: clinical
350	Quinine
110	Parasite
90	Transmission
80	Local control
70	Epidemiological theory
50	Vector eradication
	Residual insecticides
	Synthetic antimalarials
40	Liver stages
	Insecticide resistance
	Drug resistance
35	Eradication programme

Therapy substantially improved in the seventeenth century with the introduction of quinine, but otherwise the modern era began in the 1880s. As with all infectious and communicable diseases, in the late nineteenth century the field became dominated by microbiology and the causative *Plasmodium* was described in 1882. Although description of the stages of the life cycle in the mosquito soon followed, malaria was remarkable for concealing some of its parasitological secrets so that the whole life cycle, including the hypnozoite stages, took a complete century to unravel. However, malaria was equally remarkable for the very rapid translation of parasitological research to preventive

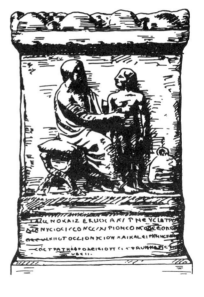

action. This was mainly due to the orientation of Ross towards practical control. On demonstrating the mosquito transmission of *Plasmodium*, Ross turned from parasitological research to field control at once and the 'mosquito theory' was put to use within a few years, with great success, particularly by Watson in Malaysia and Gorgas in Panama. The subsequent rate of malariological research steadily increased, and while the frantic pace of modern molecular biological research is a very recent phenomenon, enormous progress was made in the first half of this century in many aspects of malaria, a substantial part by workers at or on the staff of this School: Short and Garnham on the parasitology of the exo-erythrocytic stages, Christophers and Macdonald on epidemiological theory and Hamilton Fairley on clinical aspects. However, this chapter focuses on the conceptual aspects of control.

The nineteenth century saw great improvements in the control of communicable disease, chiefly as a consequence of environmental improvements. The provision of a safe piped water supply to every household was the most striking of a series of measures to improve the health of the population as a whole. This may be described as the public health approach. Environmental improvements and legislation were intended to protect all the population of a geographically defined area. Although the selection of areas might be socially determined, the goal was universal protection, both in principle and because, for the communicable diseases, to protect one's neighbour was also to help protect oneself. The public health approach (in this limited sense) to malaria is reduction in transmission, aiming to protect everyone. In this sense it relates both to Ross's view of malaria control and to the mosquito control methods for which he provided the basis. Thus in Figure 2 I identify Ross with transmission control, having as its goal an overall reduction in malaria incidence.

An alternative approach to disease control has been to seek to protect the individual. In malaria, this goes back to the use of quinine as a prophylactic and is most clearly seen today as the use of chemoprophylaxis by travellers to malarious areas and the provision of chemoprophylaxis to pregnant women in endemic areas. The aim of the first is to reduce selectively the risk to the individual traveller and of the second to protect a segment of the population seen as being at high risk of morbidity. Such a strategy has usually failed if applied to whole populations because of difficulties in maintenance and coverage. It may therefore be viewed as an approach targeted on special risk groups and can be described as a risk approach. It is more concerned with preventing death or disease than with protecting the whole community. It bears a closer relation to clinical medicine than does transmission control, and lends itself to distribution through a curative primary health care system. In Figure 2 it is therefore linked to the clinical tradition and interference with pathogenesis; it is about patients and treatment and is here put with Manson and called a risk approach.

A vaccine (for which we wait!) in normal use concerns the risk approach. It protects the immunized and only at high levels of coverage does it substantially reduce transmission through a herd effect. The exception is a gametocyte vaccine, which exerts its benefit solely through a reduction of transmission.

I have contrasted two approaches to control. How then do available methods fit into these categories? The broad public health approach of our Victorian ancestors looked to environmental control leading to a man-made landscape under careful control and a fertile economy. Into this fits species sanitation: the selective alteration of the environment to prevent breeding of the local anopheline vectors of human malaria which was so successful in areas of relatively lower vectorial capacity and especially organized plantation agriculture in the tropics. House-spraying with residual insecticides comes into the public health category, but requires rather more cooperation from the population. The use of insecticide-impregnated bednets moves closer to a risk approach, in that it transfers more responsibility for its efficacy to the actions of the user, and ability to cooperate is related to particular groups of the population. There are indeed two types of risk approach: one where the population at risk is defined by the health service ('pregnant women will be given antimalarials') and another where the risk is more a matter of perception by the patient, as in jogging to prevent cardiovascular disease or taking chemoprophylactics against malaria. Often the two types are combined, and the likelihood increases that marginal groups may selectively fail to have access to services while needing them more.

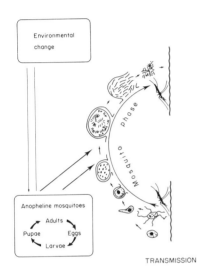

For the first two decades of this century, both environmental control of mosquito breeding and various patterns of chemotherapy were tried, and the public health approach and treatment/risk approaches were in some competition, with the French favouring chemoprophylaxis and the British vector control, as they did with sleeping sickness. Successes on the grand scale for the Panama Canal, Zambian copper belt and South Asian tea plantations made the public health approach dominant for areas where organized control of the environment was feasible, usually where there was a commercial opportunity and investment for development. The elaboration of a sophisticated species sanitation approach provided a sound basis for this. The discovery of the residual insecticidal properties of DDT changed the method of control completely, made large-scale area-wide control feasible from the 1940s (Table 4) but strengthened the predominance of transmission control, the public health approach. It also shifted any previous focus on individual protection from bites by personal action towards centralized public health efforts.

Eradication took this further still. Not only was the interruption of transmission the central goal, but chemotherapy of individuals in the consolidation phase was viewed as an attack on transmission rather than as therapy for individual benefit. There was an extreme loss of interest in the malaria patient as such (and also loss of interest in research). Eradication of malaria was treated rather as a military campaign; many of the workers were not from the health care system and the programme was usually kept separate from the remainder of the health services, at any rate until well into the consolidation phase.

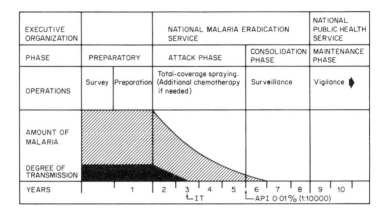

Malaria became, in a unique sense, the WHO's disease. It was chosen as a vehicle for developing the role of the WHO in the world and in some ways also carried over the approach of pre-1940 malariology, which had as its chief tool species sanitation. Control was very much in the public health tradition, with cooperation from the community necessary to permit house-spraying and active case detection, but otherwise having a minor role. Today such a description appears pejorative, though it is not intended to be so. The initial successes of the eradication policy, the lasting benefits for many countries, and the subsequent difficulties in the consolidation phase over time, are well known and need no repetition here (Table 3). The resurgence of malaria in India (Figure 3) illustrates what was seen elsewhere throughout Asia, while eradication was scarcely attempted in much of sub-Saharan Africa.

In the long and disorderly sorting out of policies during the decades of resurgence and chaos (my names; Table 4) there has been a shift towards a risk approach, in several steps. All secondary prevention amounts to a risk approach, so that treatment of the infected to prevent illness and of the ill to defer mortality is a more precisely oriented risk approach than one which focuses on population groups defined by age, pregnancy or occupation. This approach of preventing deaths and shortening illness was initially conceded with reluctance to communities otherwise unable to cope with malaria, and has gradually become more vigorously advocated by the WHO in its expert committees and their reports and follow-up groups. Much of this has been related to resolving

Table 3   Current risk of malaria in relation to past
eradication efforts in the world

Never	1300 M
Eradicated	800 M
Reduced[a]	2120 M
No control	370 M

[a] There is considerable lumping of data by countries which exaggerates
the 'reduced' category.

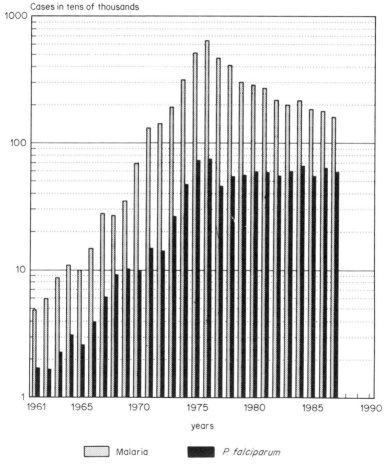

Cases in tens of thousands

Figure 3   The resurgence of malaria in India after attempts at eradication (note that the
vertical scale is logarithmic)

tensions between malaria control strategies and the primary health care concept which succeeded malaria eradication as a driving ideology at the WHO, though both ideas are now moving to more empirical approaches, partly driven by economic pressures. The move from eradication by transmission control to a risk approach to malaria has had many excellent effects. The WHO has shown an interest in the management of life-threatening malaria and the various issues related to that, and has spelled out approaches to the practical chemotherapy of malaria in the field, and this is all to the good.

There are three features of this trend that are of concern, one peculiar to malaria today, the others more general. Nobody can look at the list of available antimalarials today with any complacency: the safe drugs are rapidly becoming ineffective, and the more effective drugs are either new or relatively toxic or both, and are expensive. New drugs may well soon be followed by parasite resistance, or previously inadequately perceived toxic effects may emerge, as was the case when amodiaquine was used for prophylaxis on a larger scale. And the list of candidate new drugs is tiny. As chloroquine resistance spreads to cover Africa, what remains that is both safe and cheap? The situation cannot change overnight as the gestation period for a new drug is long — nearer a decade than a year — and few join the queue to enter.

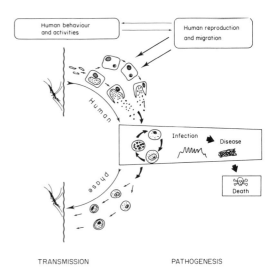

TRANSMISSION   PATHOGENESIS

Table 4   An attempt to epitomize the decades since 1930 in malaria control

	MALARIA
1940	
	CONTROL
1950	
	ERADICATION: ATTACK
1960	
	ERADICATION: CONSOLIDATION
1970	
	RESURGENCE
1980	
	CHAOS
1990	
	HOPE

The history of chemotherapy in disease control at community level is not encouraging for communicable diseases. Short-term successes have been numerous, but long-term chemoprophylaxis in Tanzania with chloroquine, and elsewhere with medicated salt, has not been effective against malaria, and campaigns against other parasites and bacterial and spirochaetal diseases have usually led to difficulties after an initially successful period, though it is too early to generalize.

The more general problem of a risk approach in malaria is that (unless the risk group is defined as the very poor and disadvantaged, which is politically unfeasible and operationally difficult) it tends to continue inequity. The very poor and disadvantaged are likely to have most difficulty in reaching health services, in paying for treatment, in coming within reach of maternal and child health clinics as mothers or as children, and generally in taking up what is on offer. The great advantage of the public health approach is that it aims at an area-wide reduction in transmission to benefit all — especially those most at risk of disease and death. Equity is thereby increased. Because vaccines have the features of both a risk approach and, at high coverage in areas of less stable malaria, of a public health approach, waiting for the vaccine becomes an impatient process! There is also need to define the community effects of those control methods which lie between a risk approach and public health, such as impregnated bednets. It may be possible by appropriate operational deployment of these to achieve much of the equity in health that results from a successful public health approach.

Whilst waiting for newer tools for control, there remains much scope for reutilization of methods that have been tested in the past, before availability of residual insecticides. No control method is free from problems and unwanted side-effects. But for any drug, insecticide or type of intervention we are most conscious of the limitations of the method used most recently. Since memories fade, there is a tendency for change, and anything new, about whose limitations and especially about whose long-term limitations we are ignorant, seems more attractive than the control methods currently in use and of whose defects we are most acutely aware.

It is more true of malaria than of any other disease that the present habit — especially in research laboratories — of only reading the literature of the last decade is completely inappropriate. The literature of malariology is unusually rich in profound work expressed in elegant and readable prose (or even poetry, in the case of Ross!). There is much of immediate relevance to conceptual understanding and to daily practice in such works as Hacketts' *Malaria in Europe*, the Tennessee Valley Authority's *Malaria control in impounded waters* and the Sergents' *Histoire d'un marais algérien*. The last century's work can inform the present and future: we need not learn the same bad lessons twice over.

In particular, the pre-insecticide era has much to teach us on environmental control of anophelines. The general level of current research in that area is much inferior in quantity and quality to earlier work. The words from *Malaria control in impounded waters* remain relevant:

> of malaria control methods the control of the mosquito vector is usually the most effective and desirable; also that this objective should be sought through use of the more permanent measures in contrast to those having temporary value or requiring repetitive application.

A view of the future

As we look forwards, speculation may be appropriate on the areas within which progress is both feasible and necessary and where what has already been done points to coherent development. It is clearly impossible to overstate the pressing need for new tools for control — for an effective vaccine against all malaria parasite species giving great and long-lasting protection at low cost even to the very young, for new, safe, inexpensive and efficacious drugs and insecticides and for sensitive, simple and cheap diagnostic tools. All these are of the first importance and will be discussed by others, so that other more epidemiological issues are discussed here.

The research scene for malaria has radically improved in the last decade and a half due to several ventures, of which the WHO/UNDP/IBRD Special Programme in Research and Training for Tropical Diseases is perhaps symbolic, with its emphasis on all the steps from basic laboratory work through to operational research, its international and collaborative nature and the participation of scientists from malaria-endemic and other countries in its management. There are many others, both bilateral and multilateral and national research programmes. At the level of tools for intervention it is appropriate that work on vaccines is balanced on a much smaller but exciting scale by the mosquito analogue: reducing the susceptibility of anopheline mosquitoes to malaria. It is an area explored before, in the 1970s, but then it was premature as not only was the breeding of malaria-resistant strains of the key mosquitoes intractable but also the general ecological fitness of selected strains presented a problem. But the availability of infectious vectors for genetic elements between insects has rightly revived this as a research area well worth exploration.

Several areas of clinical and field research deserve and are beginning to receive integrated research attention.

Rational microepidemiology

The epidemiology of malaria at the medium to large scale has appeared to be relatively well understood. Increasingly, a closer look at small areas and populations shows marked heterogeneity and results which, at any rate superficially, are difficult to understand. Even in much-studied areas such as The

Gambia there may be clear differences in endemicity between adjacent villages without obvious explanation. Methods for the detection of sporozoites in mosquitoes by means of monoclonal antibodies and new techniques for detecting genetic markers on malaria parasites, together with sensitive assays for chloroquine levels in the human population, can be combined with traditional malariological approaches to permit the reanalysis of malaria microepidemiology as has been done in Papua New Guinea. This has the potential to explain such anomalies as the occurrence of a second peak of anophelines annually in irrigated ricefields of West Africa yet without a second malaria peak. The hope is that a rational microepidemiology will permit a revision of the larger-scale epidemiological understanding; the danger is that so great a mass of detailed data may be collected as to exceed our capacity for understanding.

Without a vaccine, there must be heavy dependence on chemotherapy for the control of malarial morbidity and mortality. Drug resistance is now a massive problem, but with techniques for microassay of blood and urine levels and progress towards understanding the genetics of drug resistance by *Plasmodium*, a priority will then be to devise sophisticated methods for the surveillance of drug resistance and ones that can be used in field studies of the dynamics of resistance and the degree to which this is reversible in the absence of selection pressure (or even with counter-selection). Such information is needed for a rational decision on how far policies on drug availability can compensate for a lack of new drugs.

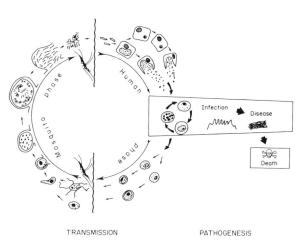

TRANSMISSION   PATHOGENESIS

Detailed community pathogenesis

A similar opportunity for using new techniques from the laboratory to gain a picture of the determinants of pathogenesis in the community is becoming available. Methods for dissection of host responses at the biochemical and immunological level are now more precise and much more sensitive (and so less invasive in their needs for blood samples) and it is possible to make progress in separating inability of human hosts to respond to certain antigens from their merely having not yet encountered them. Limitations of biologically meaningful in vitro tests for protective immunity remain. However, our understanding of the molecular biology of the pathogenetic process (and not just the immunology) is moving ahead. Whether the outcome of this work will prove operationally useful is not yet clear, but at least the way seems clear for progress towards defining the risk and possible determinants of the risk of severe disease and looking for usable markers of that risk if it be host determined.

Socioeconomic understanding of malaria in small communities

The preceding work on microepidemiology and on pathogenesis at the small community level needs to be complemented by socioeconomic and other work at the household level in terms of the perception of malaria, help-seeking behaviour if this is to be both in time to prevent severe disease and also to avoid great overuse of services, and the economic effects of malaria, especially in holoendemic areas. In a very over-simplified view (Table 5) there is perhaps great need to focus on the levels in the lower-case letters, especially the household and tissue levels, and also on microepidemiology, as well as the topics in capitals.

Issues in control strategy

In the control of malaria there has been a sequence of preferred approaches, beginning from environmental control, through insecticidal control of transmission, attempted eradication, different methods for different countries, to an emphasis on chemotherapy and early treatment through primary health care. I have suggested that different strategies fall into public health approaches, which attempt to reduce transmission for the whole community, and risk approaches, which focus on the persons most likely to die or to become severely ill. This is an over-simplification. Nevertheless, I have suggested that over time there has been a swing from total reliance on the former to very strong emphasis on the latter. Some of this emphasis has been in an attempt to move entrenched positions. Nevertheless, there is a need to keep a more even balance between these two approaches whenever possible. The appropriate balance will depend on levels of endemicity, population density and other variables. Where transmission is low

Table 5 Levels of investigation in human
malaria (see text)

COMMUNITY
Household
PATIENT
Tissue
PARASITE
Subcellular
MOLECULE

enough to give unstable malaria and in areas of denser population, environmental measures to reduce transmission will be more appropriate. Reducing transmission far enough to benefit health will be extremely difficult in rural African holoendemic malaria.

The concept of sustainable development is beginning to affect perception of options in disease control. The term is poorly defined and has to some extent been hijacked by naive environmentalists, but it has a useful function, partly to remind us that a control procedure that cannot still be maintained ten years on will be of limited value. The environment is socially constructed and needs to be

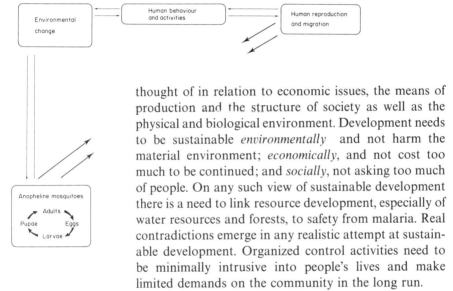

thought of in relation to economic issues, the means of production and the structure of society as well as the physical and biological environment. Development needs to be sustainable *environmentally* and not harm the material environment; *economically*, and not cost too much to be continued; and *socially*, not asking too much of people. On any such view of sustainable development there is a need to link resource development, especially of water resources and forests, to safety from malaria. Real contradictions emerge in any realistic attempt at sustainable development. Organized control activities need to be minimally intrusive into people's lives and make limited demands on the community in the long run.

In the development of water and forest resources, heavy reliance is currently placed on going through the motions of an environmental impact assessment (EIA) if international finance is needed (Figure 4). However, disease prevention issues are only indirectly addressed and action may not be taken. There is need to move towards a more positive health opportunity assessment (HOA) if adequate use is to be made of the opportunities for malaria control or prevention, both in the physical development of water resources and the provision of health care services. Preventing the malaria consequent on resource development requires specific attention.

In the control of endemic malaria elsewhere, and until new and very powerful means of intervention become available, various less than ideal methods are available. Previous methods of categorizing malarial endemicity as a guide to selecting control methods have proved inadequate. Neither the hypo-/meso-/hyper-/holoendemic categories nor the stable/unstable types give sufficient

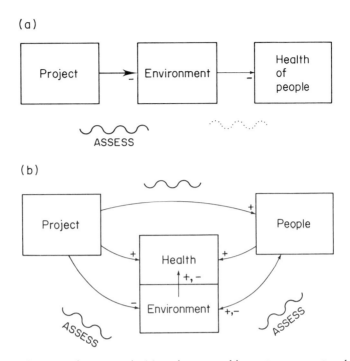

Figure 4   Diagrams of processes in (a) environmental impact assessment and (b) health
opportunity assessment

information to guide control. However, the detailed studies of epidemiology,
pathogenesis and socioeconomic aspects of malaria referred to above, combined
with environmental work on the anopheline vectors, should enable a redefined
set of epidemiological and socioeconomic types of malaria to be formulated,
which can be used in planning appropriate and sustainable malaria control.
These types of categories have sometimes been called paradigms. The aim is to
go beyond the simple stratification by parasite rate or incidence that has been
used in national malaria programmes for many years to a more rational
categorization which allows of different approaches to control. An attempt at a
broad classification is shown in Table 6.

Special attention will need to be given to focal malaria: limited areas of high
endemicity presenting particular features. Two sorts of focal malaria may be
helpfully distinguished: patches and ecotones or fringes.

Focal patches of malaria may be found in cities and in enterprises such as
mines and plantation agriculture. These patches are usually characterized by a
high population density and are the site of some organized activity, usually with
a hierarchical management. These circumstances lend themselves well to

Table 6 A broad categorization of malaria types in relation to control needs

HOLOENDEMIC
ENDEMIC
FOCAL
Patches
Ecotones
EPIDEMIC

environmental methods of malaria control and it is feasible to insist on an organized action against transmission.

The fringes between two environments, or ecotones, represent linear malaria problems. Examples are forest fringes and the edges of cities. Here circumstances are the opposite of those occurring in patches of malaria. The ecotones often move over time as the forest recedes or the city expands; the population is often highly mobile and their homes or occupations may be of dubious legality; ordered government may be deficient and the practical data needed for control scarcely available. The problems of fringe malaria may require a very flexible approach and need much further attention: they are likely to be intractable for reasons beyond the deficiency of control methods.

Manpower for control

Comparable in severity with the defects of control tools is the scarcity of trained and experienced staff. Manson's other concern, besides clinical work and research, was with training, with fitting people for the demands of tropical careers, and with the provision of those careers. The need remains, and it has become more pressing. It is a truism that malaria eradication eradicated malariologists rather than malaria; the effects of subsequent policies of integration with primary health care have been equally unintended and equally disastrous. The head of malaria in the ministry of health is almost always a doctor. Once he may have been a specialist malariologist, now he is likely to hold the job for a couple of years on his way up the ministry hierarchy. The resulting breadth of background may be an advantage; the lack of specific expertise is a disaster. The next tier down, usually entomologists, provides the continuity and technical expertise, which in the habitat biology of mosquitoes may be great, but in general the entomologist's training is even narrower than the physician's, so that the necessary breadth and depth of expertise are not found in malaria units. Team-work, though necessary, is not an adequate substitute for the multidisciplinary integration that takes place in one suitably educated and experienced person's head. The issues are sufficiently similar for other diseases transmitted by insects that vector-borne diseases can usefully form the remit for a specific group within the ministy of health, but only if the rest of the ministry do *not* see it as just a vector control unit.

Integration of operational malaria control with primary health care increases the demands for malariological expertise and the ability to communicate this expertise effectively to non-specialists. If implementation is by multipurpose workers, then their instructions and training will have to be highly focused and specific so far as malaria is concerned. The more general problems of career structure for field malariologists and other medical epidemiologists remain intractable.

Conclusion

The conclusion I reach is that, outside of sub-Saharan Africa, there is a great range of imperfect tools for malaria control, that with prudent selection and competent and diligent implementation they are capable of effecting a very substantial degree of malaria control even while we wait for a vaccine, but that this requires a breadth and depth of understanding by those in charge of planning and implementation and meticulous work by those in the field. In the last century of antimalarial work we have a wide range of methods for intervention. We have run through many approaches and techniques, but as each new one comes in we have tended to forget the previous ones. No method is useless, and inadequate application is not always a reason for rejecting a method. Although I have discussed very broad principles, the advice of Blake is more applicable to actual operations:

> He who would do good must do it in minute particulars; the general good is the cry of the charlatan

It is in the combination of the skills and methods of successive generations that good control of malaria emerges. When the insights of anthropology and education fully permeate the way in which environmental control is implemented and are not just added on as afterthoughts, and when the most sophisticated results of molecular biology are applied through appropriate simple technologies to epidemiological strategies developed decades ago, then real progress in control can be made.

I have not included sub-Saharan Africa in the above comments, even though the need is greatest there, and the comments are undoubtedly relevant to highland areas, and to the northern arid and southern temperate margins of that zone. But for the remainder of sub-Saharan Africa, while a well-deployed attack in an integrated way can have dramatic effects, especially in urban areas, the need for new tools is central. Although much action is needed, we do have to wait for the vaccine before massive success is likely. But the newer techniques of preventing bites with insecticide-impregnated bednets have been more success-ful than anticipated and are well worth exploiting, along with chemotherapy of illness, in the meantime.

Various agencies in addition to the WHO also have special skills and opportunities that can be contributed to an overall attack on the problem of malaria. Thus the World Bank is particularly well placed both to ensure that physical infrastructure reduces rather than increases malaria and to help push the health considerations in resource development down to encompass small-scale developments as well as large impoundments of water.

The most pressing intellectual challenge, requiring collaboration between researchers and operational workers, after the above combination of all (and not just recent) past experience, will be to take the rapidly growing body of detailed epidemiological understanding at the micro level and the unfolding work on molecular mechanisms of pathogenesis and so of risk, and to incorporate them, together with socioeconomic considerations, into a macro-epidemiological understanding that can be the basis of operational control programmes. Over the next few years we shall uncover a vast amount of fine detail and get precise answers to what, until recently, were feared to be imprecise questions about variation in clinical course and about inter-community variation in transmis-sion. If there is to be a scientific and rational basis for control, these will need to be incorporated into a meso- or macroepidemiological basis for realistic national plans.

Hopefully, the present decade will see a transition from chaos to hope in malaria control. Vaccines could transform the scene, but even if not, there are multiple advances taking place into all aspects of malariology. As we learn the new, we must not forget the old. As there emerge new emphases, there is still the old dilemma between Ross and Manson, between public health and risk approaches. But this is not an either/or choice but rather that of the appropriate balance. To make use of the opportunities will certainly require proper careers, education and training, and it will entail multidisciplinary activity, but with these we can look ahead with some hope even in the midst of great difficulty.

Acknowledgement

This chapter comes from the British ODA-supported Programme on Tropical Diseases Control at the LSHTM.

Clinical malaria—new problems in patient management

Kevin Marsh, Charles R.J.C. Newton, Peter A. Winstanley, J. Ben Were and
Fenella Kirkham

Kenya Medical Research Institute, Kilifi, Kenya

Introduction

The numerical aspects of malaria are staggering—over 2000 million people live
in areas of exposure and probably between 200 and 400 million cases of clinical
disease occur each year (WHO, 1989; Sturchler, 1989). Of the four species of
malaria parasites that commonly infect man only *Plasmodium falciparum* causes
significant mortality rates; at a rough estimate 90% of its associated mortality
falls on children in Africa. The 'probably' and 'rough estimates' highlight a
major problem: the dearth of epidemiological information on malaria as a
clinical disease.

It might be felt that a contribution on clinical management is of marginal
significance in a forum concerned with the larger aspects of control, and it could
be argued that clinical research largely misses the point with diseases that have
such an enormous community mortality. Reliable data are scanty but the figure
of a million childhood deaths in sub-Saharan Africa each year is probably in the
right area. Even if 90% of deaths occur in the community this still means that
around 100 000 deaths a year may occur in hospital or other treatment facilities.
The overall hospital inpatient mortality from malaria is of the order of 10%. If
the untreated mortality of this group were around 50% (a plausible estimate) it
follows that the hospital system may already be dealing with between a third
and a half of the total potentially life-threatening episodes. A reduction in
hospital mortality by improved management could lead to the avoidance of tens
of thousands of childhood deaths a year. The guestimates involved here are
admittedly wide but do not diminish the central point: that hospital-based
treatment, while a relatively small part of the total effort, may have a significant
role in control strategies as a whole.

It is important to appreciate the context in which malarial morbidity and
mortality occur. In a rural Gambian community, children aged under 5 years
had an average of one clinical attack of malaria each year and each attack
carried a 1% risk of dying (Greenwood *et al.*, 1987). There are over 100 million
children in this age group in Africa and there are therefore two broad areas of

concern: first, how to tackle the enormous load of clinical malaria at more peripheral levels; and second, how best to manage the proportionally small, but absolutely large, number of life-threatening disease episodes. The first area has been reviewed comprehensively by Breman and Campbell (1988) in the context of the African Child Survival Initiative CCCD programme for reducing malaria morbidity and mortality. They have stressed the importance of specific national malaria control units integrated into primary health care programmes. Key activities are the production of written malaria plans, standardized treatment and prevention protocols, and systems for surveillance of both the programme's operation and drug sensitivity patterns.

In the next section we consider severe clinical disease. The title of this chapter might be considered misleading as the most important problems are not new, though they may not always have been recognized. However, new possibilities are emerging for solving some of these problems and the focus of this chapter will be on severe life-threatening disease and particularly on possible options for reducing mortality.

The clinical problem

Most clinical episodes of malaria comprise a febrile illness with rather non-specific symptoms. A number of severe manifestations may supervene (see WHO, 1990, for a comprehensive review). These are listed in Table 1. Much of the detailed work on severe disease has been carried out in non-immune adults.

Table 1   Severe manifestations and complications of falciparum
malaria (from WHO, 1990, with permission)

Defining criteria of severe disease
  (1)   Cerebral malaria (unrousable coma)
  (2)   Severe normocytic anaemia
  (3)   Renal failure
  (4)   Pulmonary oedema
  (5)   Hypoglycaemia
  (6)   Circulatory collapse, shock
  (7)   Spontaneous bleeding/disseminated intravascular coagulation
  (8)   Repeated generalized convulsions
  (9)   Acidaemia/acidosis
(10)   Malarial haemoglobinuria

Other manifestations
  (1)   Impaired consciousness but rousable
  (2)   Prostration, extreme weakness
  (3)   Hyperparasitaemia
  (4)   Jaundice
  (5)   Hyperpyrexia

There are striking differences in the spectrum of severe disease in young African children. Certain features important in adults appear to be rather rare in children. These include pulmonary oedema, hepatic failure and acute renal failure. Other complications such as hypoglycaemia assume greater importance in children.

Children with severe malaria fall into three important groups: (1) cerebral malaria; (2) severe malarial anaemia; (3) others who fall short of the strict definition of cerebral malaria but who have severe features such as multiple fits, prostration and hyperparasitaemia. The overall mortality of severe inpatient malaria is around 10% (based on our experience and Brewster et al., 1990). The mortality of cerebral malaria in children has been reported to vary between 5% (Commey et al., 1980) and 38% (Guignard, 1963). Although there may be genuine differences between the various epidemiological settings the wide spread in these figures is probably due to the use of different diagnostic criteria (WHO, 1990).

Mortality is not the only problem. It is perhaps understandable that in the face of such a devastating disease as cerebral malaria emphasis has been put on the remarkable speed and completeness of recovery in survivors. However, a wide range of serious neurological sequelae have been reported, including cortical blindness, hemipareses, extrapyramidal syndromes and severe mental impairment (see Brewster et al., 1990, for review). Severe deficits occur in around 10% of survivors. It is likely that less obvious deficits are even more common. This area assumes greater importance as societies move from farming to skill-based economies, where even a minor degree of persistent clumsiness may be a major problem for an adult. The sheer number of cases of severe malaria may mean that inapparent neurological deficit is a large unrecognized public health problem.

How much of the mortality is preventable even in theory? Over 50% of deaths due to cerebral malaria occur later than 12 hours after admission to hospital. Although even early deaths may be avoided by intervention, for example correction of hypoglycaemia or acidosis (see below), it is likely that later deaths are most amenable to prevention. One might therefore reasonably ask why any child who survives 12 hours should die, given that peak concentrations of antimalarials can be achieved in one or two hours; thereafter the situation should, in theory at least, be improving. There are two main possibilities for the development of novel management: (1) new regimens of antimalarial drugs; (2) therapy based on the specific pathophysiology of malarial disease.

Antimalarial drugs and severe malaria

It is only the last few years that have seen the application of rigorous pharmacological principles to the design of regimens for the treatment of severe malaria. The major questions in Africa are: what is the optimum way to use quinine; and do any other parenteral drugs have a significant advantage over quinine?

There has been considerable controversy over the use of a loading dose of quinine. Its use is supported by the demonstration of the safety of such regimens (White et al., 1983b) and by the recent finding that clearance of the bulk of the parasites is correlated with the area under the concentration versus time curve for quinine in the first 24 hours of treatment (Pasvol et al., 1991). The demonstration that 12-hourly doses of drug can achieve as good profiles as 8-hourly (Waller et al., 1990; Pasvol et al., 1991) and that the intramuscular route gives profiles comparable with those obtained by intravenous administration (Waller et al., 1990; Mansoor et al., 1990; Pasvol et al., 1991) is of real practical importance for the management of severe disease in situations where there are shortages of skilled staff.

While it must be right to optimize drug regimens, to date there is no clear evidence of major reductions in mortality from such an approach. There are two possible reasons: first, it may be that quinine is already doing the best it can; second, the tools that we have for comparing alternative drug regimens in severe malaria are inadequate. They have been developed in the context of non-severe malaria and are heavily dependent on such parameters as time to parasite clearance. In severe disease, what counts is the effect on mortality and serious morbidity; there is therefore a need to develop alternative end-points for therapeutic trials (White and Krishna, 1989). Ultimately, the major question is whether a particular regimen prevents more deaths. This problem requires studies of a size beyond the capability of most research centres. It will be necessary to build up the capacity to carry out multicentre trials in Africa if we are ever to have a clear-cut answer to these important questions.

Would the use of alternative antimalarials in place of, or in addition to, quinine improve outcome? At presentation there are two populations of parasites to consider: the ones you can see — immature stages in the peripheral circulation — and the ones you cannot see — mature parasites sequestered in deep vascular beds.

There is a natural tendency to concentrate on the parasites that can be seen, whereas it is the second population that is causing the immediate damage. After the institution of specific antimalarial drugs the size of the peripheral population of parasites usually stays constant or even rises for up to 24 hours, then goes into a decline, the timing and rate of which is often used as an outcome measure. It is, however, unlikely that the disappearance of parasites from the peripheral circulation represents a direct effect of the drug on these parasites. Quinine acts preferentially on mature parasites in the second half of the cycle, i.e. those that are already sequestered. Incubation of young ring-stage parasites with quinine in vitro had minimal effect on their development up to the stage when they would normally sequester, and they behaved normally in an in vitro model of sequestration (Marsh, unpublished observation). We have recently obtained preliminary evidence that this response occurs *in vivo*. Parasite viability during treatment with quinine, as judged by their ability to mature and cytoadhere, remained normal until the time of parasite disappearance from the peripheral circulation (Watkins *et al.*, in preparation). Thus the parasite clearance curve during treatment combines two components: the normal movement out of the circulation of the visible parasite population; and the curtailment of the appearance of new parasites from the sequestered population. In non-severe malaria it matters little that the circulating population of parasites remains viable and functionally active for up to 24 hours after the start of treatment, but in severe malaria further sequestration in compromised tissue beds may be disastrous. This sequestration could explain some of the sudden deaths between 12 and 36 hours in cerebral malaria.

There is therefore a potential role for antimalarial drugs capable of acting quickly on young parasites and preventing their sequestration. Derivatives of the Chinese herbal remedy qinghaosu may do this (Qinghaosu Antimalaria Coordinating Research Group, 1979). In the *in vitro* experiments referred to above, the derivatives were able to arrest maturation and prevent cytoadherence. Progress in looking critically at these drugs outside China has been woefully slow.

If killing a proportion of the total parasite population as large and as quickly as possible is important in severe disease it may be that the ideal drug regimen will include a combination of several antimalarials with different points of action in the parasite life cycle. However, the possibility that rapid parasite death may itself have pathological consequences should be borne in mind.

It may be that killing the parasites is not enough and that therapy needs to be specifically targeted at the pathophysiological processes of severe disease. In the following sections we consider some of the processes which may be important in severe malaria in the light of current management problems and potential new approaches.

Parasite sequestration

The characteristic histopathological feature of cerebral malaria is the packing of the small vessels of the brain with erythrocytes containing mature parasites (MacPherson *et al.*, 1985). Clearly, specific reversal of massive cerebral sequestration could be beneficial. Although most antimalarial drugs act on mature parasites, it is unlikely that they lead to early release from the vascular beds as this has not been observed clinically and does not occur in *in vitro* models (Marsh, unpublished observations). There are a number of potential lines of attack. First, immune individuals produce antibodies capable of binding specifically to the infected red cell surface and interfering with the adhesion process (Udeinya *et al.*, 1983). Infusion of immune sera in a primate host of *P. falciparum* leads to rapid release of sequestered parasites (David *et al.* 1983).

Preliminary observations in human patients indicated that antibodies capable of blocking cytoadherence *in vitro* had no parasite-releasing effect when passively infused as part of therapeutic blood transfusions (Marsh, unpublished). The use of hyperimmune serum is being investigated in a trial in Malawi. If this line shows any promise there is the potential of developing more specific immunological therapy using monospecific or monoclonal antibodies.

An alternative strategy would be based on a detailed understanding of the process of infected red cell cytoadherence which underlies sequestration. To date three candidate molecules have been identified for the role of endothelial receptors: thrombospondin (Roberts et al., 1985), CD36 (Barnwell et al., 1985) and intracellular adhesion molecule 1 (ICAM 1) (Berendt et al., 1989). There may well be others yet to be discovered. The role of these receptors in specific anatomical sites remains to be established but progress in identifying the exact molecular mechanisms of binding is well advanced. For instance, in the case of ICAM 1, fragments of the whole molecule have been made which can interfere with binding (Berendt, personal communication) and this kind of approach will open the way for the design of specific competitors with the potential for use as therapeutic agents.

Hypoglycaemia

It is only in the past eight years that hypoglycaemia has been widely recognized as a major complication of severe malaria needing prompt and careful management. This is perhaps surprising as hypoglycaemia is a feature of many animal models of malaria (Sadun et al., 1965), was sporadically reported in children with malaria (Hendrikse, 1987) and has clinical manifestations which include coma, fitting and decerebrate posturing, i.e. the features of cerebral malaria. In adult Thais, 8% of patients with severe malaria were hypoglycaemic. This was a problem particularly in pregnant women, 50% of whom were hypoglycaemic (White et al., 1983a). Hypoglycaemia is even more common in African children, occurring in 32% and 23% of cases of cerebral malaria reported in The Gambia (White et al., 1987) and Malawi (Molyneux et al., 1989), respectively. Hypoglycaemia is an important prognostic factor, being associated with a greater than 40% mortality in cerebral malaria compared with around 7% in cerebral malaria cases which remained normoglycaemic (Brewster et al., 1990; Molyneux et al., 1989). The pathogenesis is complex and involves both a reduction in supply due to inhibition of gluconeogenesis and an increase in demand due to obligatory utilization by parasites. In Thai patients hypoglycaemia was accompanied by a hyperinsulinaemic state with high concentrations of C-peptide, alanine and lactate (White et al., 1983a). This situation is particularly associated with treatment with quinine, which is a potent stimulator of insulin production by islet cells. The situation in African children is less clear; quinine-related hypoglycaemia has been reported in Zaire (Okitolonda *et al.*, 1987) and Madagascar (Robin *et al.*, 1989). However, in two carefully documented series in The Gambia and Malawi (White *et al.*, 1987; Taylor *et al.*, 1988) there was no evidence of a hyperinsulinaemic state and hypoglycaemia occurred in the absence of prior treatment with quinine.

Recently doubt has been cast on the specificity of the connection between severe malaria and hypoglycaemia (Kawo *et al.*, 1990). While it is important to realize that hypoglycaemia may be a feature of many severe childhood illnesses, there is no doubt that the frequency and nature of hypoglycaemia in severe malaria are such as to warrant its being regarded as a specific and important complication.

Correction of hypoglycaemia in cerebral malaria rarely leads to an immediate improvement in the level of consciousness of the child, indicating that it is not the primary cause of the condition. However, it is essential that this observation does not lead to any sense of therapeutic nihilism, as whatever other therapeutic manoeuvres are introduced they will not be able to show their true effect in children who are allowed to remain hypoglycaemic. Worries have been expressed that correction of hypoglycaemia with dextrose could lead to a rebound worsening of lactic acidosis and could remove a putative protective effect of hypoglycaemia in anoxic brain damage (White, 1986). There is no evidence that either of these possibilities is important in practice and there is plenty of evidence to suggest that prolonged severe hypoglycaemia carries a grave threat of death or persistent neurological deficit.

Blood glucose must be measured on admission and regularly thereafter in any child with any feature of severe malaria and in all pregnant women with malaria. Hypoglycaemia should be treated vigorously by correction with 50% dextrose and the likelihood of recurrence countered by repeated monitoring of blood glucose and a continuous infusion of 10% dextrose if necessary. In the absence of the means to measure blood sugar, hypoglycaemia should be assumed in any comatose child with malaria and treated appropriately. The role of glucagon in the acute management of hypoglycaemia in children with severe malaria has not been fully assessed. In Thai adults the glucose response was often poor (White *et al.*, 1983a), and this has been our experience in children. The insulin-releasing effect of glucagon argues against its use if there is the possibility of a hyperinsulinaemic state. The somatostatin analogue SMS201/995 is effective in correcting hyperinsulinaemia (Phillips *et al.*, 1986); however, this treatment is unlikely to have wide application as most African children are not hyperinsulinaemic and the drug is not generally available.

It is worrying that in many places awareness of hypoglycaemia in malaria is low and attempts at treatment are often inadequate. It is a high priority to ensure that staff managing malaria are aware of the nature and importance of hypoglycaemia in severe malaria and have the means available to detect and treat it promptly.

Lactic acidosis

Elevated levels of lactate in the blood and cerebrospinal fluid (CSF) are common in cerebral malaria in children (Molyneux *et al.*, 1989) and adults (White *et al.*, 1985) and are higher in fatal cases than in survivors. Lactic acidosis is often but not always associated with hypoglycaemia. As with hypoglycaemia, mechanisms are complex and probably involve both accumulation due to host and parasite anaerobic glycolysis, and reduced hepatic clearance. Lactic acidosis is both a marker of severity and a pathophysiological risk factor in its own right.

It is important to take a very aggressive approach to the management of children with severe acidosis. It is difficult to gain peripheral venous access — central access should be established immediately. Similarly there should be no hesitation in deciding to intubate and hand ventilate while the situation is stabilized. The most important aspects of management are prompt and effective treatment with antimalarials, correction of fluid and electrolyte imbalances, correction of hypoglycaemia, improvement of oxygenation, and treatment of concurrent infection. There is no consensus on the use of bicarbonate. Although logical to correct pH, the use of bicarbonate may lead to a concomitant fall in intracellular and cerebral pH (Bradley and Semple, 1962) and may also necessitate giving an undesirable hyperosmotic load if 50% dextrose is also required at the same time. Our own practice is to rely on very vigorous general management and the use of bicarbonate if the pH falls below 7.1. A number of therapeutic approaches have been tried in lactic acidosis in other settings but few have been successful. One potentially interesting option is the use of dichloracetate, an inducer of pyruvate dehydrogenase, which will lead to the increased utilization of lactate. In a rodent model of malaria, dichloracetate led to a significant attenuation of the rise in lactate and also caused a reduction in the fall in pH associated with hyperparasitaemia (Holloway *et al.*, 1991). Given the seriousness of the situation it would be appropriate to investigate the potential use of this compound in patients with severe lactic acidosis.

Intracranial hypertension

Raised intracranial pressure has not generally been considered to play a role in the pathogenesis of cerebral malaria. In non-immune adults with cerebral malaria CSF opening pressures at lumbar puncture were usually in the normal range and were lower in fatal cases (Warrell *et al.*, 1986). Nonetheless, some workers have claimed that children with cerebral malaria may have raised intracranial pressure (Commey *et al.*, 1980; Thapa *et al.*, 1988) and we were prompted to investigate this possibility in the light of accumulating evidence for a role of raised intracranial pressure in a wide range of encephalopathies of childhood (Goitein *et al.*, 1983).

CSF opening pressures in Kenyan children with cerebral malaria were always outside the normal range for age, and 30% had very high pressure (Newton *et al.*, 1991). These findings, while novel, do not in themselves establish that intracranial hypertension plays any role in the pathogenesis of severe disease. Potential mechanisms for such an effect are the production of global or local ischaemia by the ensuing reduction in cerebral perfusion pressure and the herniation of cranial contents as a direct result of the rise in pressure. Retrospective analysis of detailed neurological examinations in 60 children with cerebral malaria showed that all of the 12 children who died had clinical evidence of herniation syndromes, compared with 35% of the survivors. Furthermore 7 out of the 12 fatal cases but none of the survivors had evidence of rostro-caudal progression in the signs of herniation. Taken together these findings argue strongly for a role for intracranial hypertension in the pathogenesis of severe malaria in African children.

Evidence from studies in adults suggests that neither cerebral oedema nor hydrocephalus are features of cerebral malaria (Looaresuan *et al.*, 1983). We propose that in severe malaria the sequestered mass of infected red cells acts as a (diffuse) space-occupying lesion and increases cerebral blood volume. As cerebral blood flow does not appear to be reduced (Warrell *et al.*, 1988) this increased blood volume will lead to a rise in intracranial pressure. Furthermore, sequestered mature parasites release large amounts of lactate, a powerful vasodilator, which may compound the problem. In such a situation cerebral function may be poised on a knife edge, where a critical reduction in cerebral perfusion pressure may lead to ischaemic damage and also to further rise in intracranial pressure (Rosner and Becker, 1984). This scenario could account for many of the clinical features of severe malaria.

The recognition and treatment of intracranial hypertension has become an important part of the management of many childhood encephalopathies and it is now important to assess the roles of potential therapies, including osmotic diuretics to lower intracranial pressure, and the possible use of inotropes to maintain cerebral perfusion pressures. Exciting though these prospects are, it is essential that such approaches are not adopted before there has been a clear demonstration of their likely benefit.

The findings also have practical implications for the immediate management of comatose children with malaria. In such cases lumbar puncture (LP) is considered mandatory to exclude the possibility of meningitis (WHO, 1990). The risks of carrying out an LP in the presence of raised intracranial pressure are not clear. Many clinicians worry about the possibility of coning and we have certainly seen this happen following LP in malaria. However, it is not at all certain that this is cause and effect. Our own practice is now to delay LP until the patient is neurologically stable and to cover the possibility of meningitis in the interim with chloramphenicol. When LP is performed it would be prudent to have an osmotic diuretic available in case opening pressure is very high. LP should certainly be avoided in the presence of localizing signs of brainstem abnormalities.

Tumour necrosis factor

It has been proposed that many of the clinical features of malaria are mediated by host cytokines secreted in response to parasite infection (Clark *et al.*, 1981). Most attention has focused on tumour necrosis factor (TNF), a macrophage product with important roles in many host defence functions (Beutler and Cerami, 1987). The proposal is based on a large weight of evidence on the effects of TNF *in vitro* and *in vivo*, particularly its ability to induce some of the features of malaria in a variety of model systems (Clark, 1987) and the prevention of these features in experimental rodent malarias by the use of antibodies to both TNF and other mediators in the pathway to TNF release (Grau *et al.*, 1989). Circulating TNF levels are raised in the sera of malaria patients (Scuderi *et al.*, 1986). In both African children (Grau *et al.*, 1989; Kwiatowski *et al.*, 1990) and non-immune Europeans (Kern *et al.*, 1989) with *P. falciparum* infections, circulating TNF levels were significantly higher in cases with severe complications. Furthermore, in children with cerebral malaria TNF levels were predictive of a fatal outcome.

The relevance of these observations to clinical management depends on whether TNF is a marker of severity or, as seems more likely, directly involved in pathogenesis. The timing of events will also be important; for instance, TNF is able to upregulate expression of a number of endothelial surface receptors including ICAM 1 (Berendt *et al.*, 1989) and this may be an early event in the chain leading to cerebral sequestration. However, it is unlikely that, in this case, an intervention aimed at TNF would improve the situation once coma was established. Alternatively the deleterious effects of TNF may be closely dependent on its continuing release. There is no clear evidence on this, though it might be argued that the rapid decline in TNF levels of survivors but not those who subsequently die supports this scenario (Kwiatowski *et al.*, 1990).

The most obvious intervention is the use of anti-TNF antibodies. These have proved effective in preventing or abrogating TNF-mediated pathology in some experimental systems, including endotoxic shock (Tracey *et al.*, 1987) and a murine model of cerebral malaria (Grau *et al.*, 1987). However, in these cases success depended on the administration of anti-TNF antibodies at an earlier point in the disease than would be practicable for most patients who develop severe malaria. The only way to get a clear answer in human malaria will be to perform a controlled trial. The real importance of the emerging picture of the role of TNF and other cytokines in the pathogenesis of malaria may be in directing attention to new therapeutic approaches to be used early in the illness to prevent progression to severe disease.

Convulsions in severe malaria

Convulsions are a common feature of malaria. In adults, almost by definition, they indicate that the patient has cerebral malaria. In children the situation is rather different because of the susceptibility between the ages of 6 months and 6 years to so-called febrile fits. The view that fits in children who do not have cerebral malaria are febrile fits, simply reflecting the fact that malaria is such a common cause of fever, has been challenged (Hendrikse, 1987). Preliminary analysis of our experience suggests that in many cases these apparently benign fits are a specific feature of malaria and carry significant risk of progression to more severe disease. Over 80% of children with cerebral malaria in Africa convulse. Fitting carries a real risk of aspiration, probably an important avoidable and under-recorded cause of death in cerebral malaria. The importance of fitting, particularly prolonged or repeated episodes, in further compromising cerebral function in an encephalopathy is not well established but there are several potential mechanisms, including exacerbation of intracranial hypertension by associated alterations in cerebrovascular control (Minns and Brown, 1978) and metabolic damage in areas of seizure activity. There are therefore good theoretical reasons to believe that prevention of fitting following admission is desirable.

The only drug likely to be of practical use in the tropics, on grounds of cost, safety and length of action, is phenobarbitone. Low-dose intramuscular phenobarbitone (3.5 mg/kg) is reported to prevent fits in adult Thais with cerebral malaria (White et al., 1988). This is a surprising result as the predicted blood levels with the dose used would be well below those normally regarded as necessary for an anticonvulsant effect, raising the possibility that subjects with malaria are particularly sensitive to the effects of phenobarbitone. It has been recommended that the same approach be adopted in children (White et al., 1988; Phillips and Solomon, 1990). In a preliminary dose-finding study we found that 10 mg/kg (i.e. three times the effective dose in adults) was without either protective or toxic effects in Kenyan children with cerebral malaria. It is therefore a high priority to establish a safe and effective prophylactic regimen. In the interim, measures to reduce the likelihood of fits and their consequences should be rigorously applied: the temperature of children should be kept as close to normal as possible by the use of tepid sponging and fanning and the regular, rather than intermittent, use of paracetamol given rectally or by nasogastric tube. All children who are comatosed should have a nasogastric tube inserted and gastric contents aspirated. Fits should be treated aggressively and terminated with either intravenous diazepam or intramuscular paraldehyde. Alternatively both drugs can be given rectally. Status epilepticus is an indication for the careful use of intravenous phenytoin.

Anaemia

Severe anaemia is a major life-threatening complication. A proportion of cases present with severe anaemia (haemoglobin less than 5 g/dl), low-to-moderate parasitaemias and are not in heart failure. Management comprises effective clearance of parasites. A particular trap is that these children may appear quite well; but if chloroquine is used it is essential that they are followed closely to ensure complete clearance, because drug failure may lead to a rapid and disastrous deterioration. Although malaria is reported to cause varying degrees of marrow dysfunction there is usually a brisk reticulocytosis and rise in haemoglobin once the parasites are cleared. If this does not occur the use of haematinics is dictated by the clinical findings and a knowledge of the iron and folate status of the community from which the child comes. It has been suggested that children given iron in endemic areas may be at increased risk of developing clinical malaria (Smith *et al.*, 1989). There is no consensus on this and the decision as to whether such children should receive prophylactic cover will be heavily influenced by resources and drug sensitivity patterns.

A more acute management problem is presented by those children with malaria, anaemia and heart failure. The management is replacement of blood and the use of diuretics, and although this requires extreme care there are no problems specific to malaria. The major clinical problem is how to identify those children that do need transfusion and to avoid unnecessary transfusion in others. Transfusion carries risks both of HIV transmission (Nguyen-Dinh *et al.*, 1987) and of precipitating worsening failure and sudden death. Recommendations that rely on a set level of haemoglobin or haematocrit inevitably lead to more children being transfused than is necessary. There are two clear priorities. First, a general requirement is to ensure the best possible screening of blood for transfusion. If there is any doubt, it is worth trying to ensure that blood is donated by an elderly relative who may be in a lower risk group for HIV than other potential donors. Secondly, clear and realistic guidelines, for use at all levels of health services capable of transfusing children, should be developed for identifying children requiring transfusion, and standard protocols should be adopted to avoid over-transfusion.

Conclusions

Several priorities have been identified, some of which relate to rather general points that are not strictly problems in clinical management but which nonetheless are important when considering the role of treatment in malaria control programmes. A priority here is the refocusing in both research and operational areas on clinical disease. It is important to ensure that the large infrastructures that exist in many countries collect data that are relevant to the current challenge rather than continue in the tracks set when eradication dominated the thoughts of malariologists. A second general priority is the establishment wherever possible of clear-cut guidelines to the management of malaria for health personnel at all levels. The comprehensive WHO publication is a landmark, but we have yet to find a doctor in an African district hospital who has seen a copy; indeed most researchers read it in full only when preparing review articles. It should be recognized that most of the important management decisions are taken by cadres other than doctors. It should also be recognized that in many countries an enormous amount of treatment of malaria takes place out of the government health services and this sector must also be targeted for education.

The second group of priorities relate to research. Nothing could be less helpful than a large amount of inconclusive research, interesting though some of the results may be. The problem of appropriate end-points for clinical trials in severe malaria has been highlighted. Also important is the establishment of clinical research networks to allow standardized multicentre trials when there are major questions to answer.

We have summarized areas in which advances in the understanding of the disease are opening new prospects for clinical management. Clearly some of these are more speculative than others; if specific competitors of cytoadherence are a possibility, they are some years away. In contrast, there is every prospect of clear answers on important questions such as the role of alternative anti-malarials, the prophylaxis of fitting or the management of intracranial hypertension. As always, the greatest challenge will be to translate the results of research into practice — easy to say and hard to do. If it can be done there is the real possibility of avoiding tens of thousands of deaths due to malaria each year in Africa.

References

Barnwell JW, Ockenhouse CF and Knowles DM (1985) Monoclonal antibody OKM5 inhibits the in vitro binding of *Plasmodium falciparum* infected erythrocytes to monocytes, endothelial and C32 melanoma cells. *Journal of Immunology, 135*, 3494–3497

Berendt AR, Simmons DL, Tansey J, Newbold CI and Marsh K (1989) Intracellular adhesion molecule-1 is an endothelial receptor for a cytoadherence ligand on *Plasmodium falciparum* infected erythrocytes. *Nature, 341*, 57–59

Beutler B and Cerami A (1987) Cachectin: more than a tumour necrosis factor. *New England Journal of Medicine, 316*, 379–385

Breman JG and Campbell CC (1988) Combating severe malaria in African children. *Bulletin of the World Health Organization, 66*, 611–620

Brewster DR, Kwiatkowski D and White NJ (1990) Neurological sequelae of cerebral malaria in children. *Lancet, 336*, 1039–1043

Bradley RD and Semple SJG (1962) Comparison of certain acid–base characteristics of arterial blood, jugular venous blood and CSF in man and effects on them of some acute and chronic acid base disturbances. *Journal of Physiology, 160*, 381–391

Clark IA (1987) Monokines and lymphokines in malarial pathology. *Annals of Tropical Medicine and Parasitology, 81*, 577–585

Clark IA, Virelizier JL, Carswell EA and Wood PR (1981) Possible importance of macrophage derived mediators in acute malaria. *Infection and Immunity, 32*, 1058–1066

Commey JCC, Mills-Tetteh D and Phillips BJ (1980) Cerebral malaria in Accra, Ghana. *Ghana Medical Journal, 14*, 68–72

David PH, Hommel M, Miller LH, Udeinya IJ and Oligino LD (1983) Parasite sequestration in *Plasmodium falciparum* malaria: spleen and antibody modulation of cytoadherence of infected erythrocytes. *Proceedings of the National Academy of Sciences USA*, 80, 5075–5079

Goiten KH, Amit YJ and Mussa FH (1983) Intracranial pressure in central nervous system infections and cerebral ischaemia of infancy. *Archives of Disease in Childhood*, 58, 184–186

Grau GE, Fajard LF, Piguet PF, Allet B, Lambert PH and Vassalli (1987) Tumour necrosis factor/cachectin as an essential mediator in murine cerebral malaria. *Science*, 237, 1210–1212

Grau GE, Pignet PF, Vassalli and Lambert PH (1989) Tumour necrosis factor and other cytokines in cerebral malaria: experimental and clinical data. *Immunological Reviews*, 112, 49–69

Greenwood BM, Bradley AK, Greenwood AM, Byass P, Jammeh K, Marsh K, Tulloch S, Oldfield FSJ and Hayes R (1987) Mortality and morbidity from malaria among children in a rural area of the Gambia, West Africa. *Transactions of the Royal Society of Tropical Medicine and Hygiene*, 81, 478–486

Guignard J (1963) Le paludisme pernicieux du nourrisson et de l'enfant. Considerations cliniques, prognostiques et therapeutiques. À propos de 130 cas observé eu zone d'endemie palustre. *Annales de Pediatrie*, 43, 646–656

Hendrikse RG (1987) Malaria and child health. *Annals of Tropical Medicine and Parasitology*, 81, 499–509

Holloway PA, Krishma S and White NJ (1991) *Plasmodium berghei:* lactic acidosis and hypoglycaemia in a rodent model of severe malaria—effects of glucose, quinine and dichloracetate. *Experimental Parasitology* (in press)

Kawo NG, Msengi AE, Sawi ABM, Chuura LM, Alberti KGMM and MacLarty DG (1990) Specificity of hypoglycaemia for cerebral malaria in children. *Lancet, ii*, 454–457

Kern P, Hemmer CJ, Gruss HJ and Dietrich M (1989) Elevated tumour necrosis factor alpha and interleukin 6 serum levels as markers for complicated *Plasmodium falciparum* malaria. *American Journal of Medicine*, 87, 139–143

Kwiatkowski D, Hill AVS, Sambou I, Thumasi P, Castracane J, Manogue K, Cerami A, Brewster D and Greenwood BM (1990) TNF concentrations in fatal cerebral, non-fatal cerebral and uncomplicated *Plasmodium falciparum* malaria. *Lancet*, 336, 1201–1204

Looareesuan S, Warrell DA, White NJ, Sutherasamai P, Chanthavanich P, Sundaraveg K, Juel-Jensen BE, Bunnag D and Harinasuta T (1983) Do patients with cerebral malaria have cerebral oedema? A computed tomographic study. *Lancet, i*, 434–437

Mansoor SM, Taylor TE, McGrath CS, Edwards G, Ward SA, Wirima JJ and Molyneux ME (1990) The safety and kinetics of intramuscular quinine in Malawian children with moderately severe falciparum malaria. *Transactions of the Royal Society of Tropical Medicine and Hygiene*, 84, 482–487

MacPherson GG, Warrell MJ, White NJ, Looareesuan S and Warrell DA (1985) Human cerebral malaria: a quantitative ultrastructural analysis of parasitised erythrocyte sequestration. *American Journal of Pathology*, 119, 385–401

Minns RA and Brown JK (1978) Intracranial pressure changes associated with child-hood seizures. *Developmental Medicine and Child Neurology*, 20, 561–569

Molyneux ME, Taylor TE, Wirima JJ and Borgstein A (1989) Clinical features and prognostic indicators in paediatric cerebral malaria: a study of 131 comatose Malawian children. *Quarterly Journal of Medicine (New Series)*, 71, No. 265, 441–459

Newton CRJC, Kirkham FJ, Winstanley PA, Pasvol G, Peshu N, Warrell DA and Marsh K (1991) Raised intracranial pressure in African children with cerebral malaria. *Lancet* (in press)

Okitolonda W, Delacollette C, Mullengrean M and Henquin JC (1987) High incidence of hypoglycaemia in African patients treated with intravenous quinine for severe malaria. *British Medical Journal*, 295, 716–718

Pasvol G, Newton CRJC, Winstanley PA, Watkins WM, Peshu NM, Were JBO, Marsh K and Warrell DA (1991) Quinine treatment of severe falciparum malaria in African children: a randomized comparison of three regimens. *American Journal of Tropical Medicine and Hygiene* (in press)

Phillips RE and Solomon T (1990) Cerebral malaria in children. *Lancet*, ii, 1355–1360

Phillips RE, Warrell DA, Looareesuan S et al. (1986) Effectiveness of SMS 201–995, a synthetic long acting somatostatin analogue in treatment of quinine induced hyperinsulinaemia. *Lancet*, i, 713–716

Qinghaosu Antimalaria Coordinating Research Group (1979) Antimalarial studies on qinghaosu. *Chinese Medical Journal*, 92, 811–816

Roberts DD, Sherwood JA, Spitalnik SL, Panton LJ, Howard RJ, Dixit VM, Frazier WA, Miller LH and Ginsberg V (1985) Thrombospondin binds falciparum malaria parasitised erythrocytes and may mediate cytoadherence. *Nature*, 318, 64–66

Robin X, Le Bras J and Coulanger P (1989) Hypoglycemies severes au cours d'access pernicieux à *Plasmodium falciparum* traités par la quinine (étude sur 110 cas). *Bulletin de la Société de la Pathologie Exotique*, 82, 476–481

Rosner MJ and Becker DP (1984) Origin and evolution of plateau waves. *Journal of Neurosurgery*, 60, 312–324

Sadun EH, Williams JS, Meroney FC and Hutt G (1965) Pathophysiology of *Plasmodium berghei* infections in mice. *Experimental Parasitology*, 17, 272–304

Scuderi P, Steriling KE, Lam KS, Finley PR, Ryan KJ, Pam CG, Petersen E, Shymen DJ and Salmon SE (1986) Raised serum levels of tumour necrosis factor in parasitic infections. *Lancet*, ii, 1364–1365

Sturchler D (1989) How much malaria is there worldwide? *Parasitology Today*, 5, 39

Taylor TE, Molyneux ME, Wirima JJ, Fletcher KA and Morris K (1988) Blood glucose levels in Malawian children before and during the administration of intravenous quinine for severe falciparum malaria. *New England Journal of Medicine*, 319, 1040–1047

Thapa BR, Marwcha RK, Kumar L and Mehta S (1988) Cerebral malaria in children: therapeutic considerations. *Indian Paediatrics*, 25, 61–65

Tracey KJ, Fong Y, Hesse DG, Manogue KR, Lee DT, Kuo GC, Lowry F and Cerami A (1987) Anti-cachectin/TNF monoclonal antibodies prevent septic shock during lethal bacteraemia. *Nature*, 330, 662–664

Udeinya LJ, Miller LH, McGregor IA and Jensen JB (1983) *Plasmodium falciparum* strain specific antibody blocks binding of infected erythrocytes to amelanotic melanoma cells. *Nature*, 303, 429–431

Waller D, Krishna S, Craddock C, Brewster D, Jammeh A, Kwiatokwski D, Karbwang J, Molunto P, and White NJ (1990) The pharmacokinetic properties of intramuscular quinine in Gambian children with severe falciparum malaria. *Transactions of the Royal Society of Tropical Medicine and Hygiene*, 84, 488–491

Warrell DA, Looareesuan S, Phillips RE, White NJ, Warrell MJ, Areekul S and Tharavanij S (1986) Function of the blood–cerebrospinal fluid barrier in human cerebral malaria: rejection of the permeability hypothesis. *American Journal of Tropical Medicine and Hygiene*, 35, 882–887

Warrell DA, White NJ, Veall N, Looareesuan S, Chanthavanich P, Phillips, RE, Karbwang J and Pongpaew P (1988) Cerebral anaerobic glycolysis and reduced cerebral oxygen transport in human cerebral malaria. *Lancet*, ii, 534–538

White NJ (1986) Pathophysiology. *Clinics in Tropical Medicine and Communicable Diseases*, 1, 55–90

White NJ and Krishna S (1989) Treatment of malaria; some considerations and limitations of the current methods of assessment. *Transactions of the Royal Society of Tropical Medicine and Hygiene, 83,* 767–777

White NJ, Warrell DA, Chanthavanich P, Looaresnwan S, Warrell MJ, Krishna S, Williamson DH and Turner RC (1983a) Severe hypoglycaemia and hyperinsulinaemia in falciparum malaria. *New England Journal of Medicine, 369,* 61–66

White NJ, Looaresnwan S, Warrell DA, Warrell MJ, Chanthavanich P, Bunnag D and Harinasuta, T (1983b) Quinine loading dose in cerebral malaria. *American Journal of Tropical Medicine and Hygiene, 32,* 1–5

White NJ, Warrell DA, Looaresnwan S, Chanthavanich P, Phillips RE and Pongpaew P (1985) Pathophysiologic and prognostic significance of cerebrospinal-fluid lactate in cerebral malaria. *Lancet, i,* 776–778

White NJ, Miller KD, Marsh K, Berry CD, Turner RC, Williamson DH and Brown J (1987) Hypoglycaemia in African children with severe malaria. *Lancet, i,* 708–711

White NJ, Looaresnwan S, Phillips RE, Chanthavanich P and Warrell DA (1988) Single dose phenobarbitone prevents convulsions in cerebral malaria. *Lancet, ii,* 64–66

WHO (1989) *Weekly Epidemiological Record, 32,* 241–247

WHO (1990) Severe and complicated malaria. *Transactions of the Royal Society of Tropical Medicine and Hygiene, 84,* (Suppl.), 1–65

WORKSHOP REPORT AND RECOMMENDATIONS
RAPPORTEUR: PHUC NGUYEN-DIN

Patients dying with malaria in hospitals probably represent only a minute fraction of all patients dying of the disease, especially in Africa. For example, in a rural community in The Gambia in 1982–1983, of 25 children under 7 years old dying of an illness that was probably malaria, 23 died at home, 2 died in a dispensary, and none died in hospital (Greenwood *et al.,* 1987). In Togo in 1989 reported hospital deaths and population-based data suggest that only one in 31–35 malaria deaths occurred in hospitals (Nguyen Dinh, unpublished results). Thus, prevention, recognition and treatment of severe malaria at peripheral levels, in the homes, health posts and dispensaries, constitute a priority approach to the management of clinical malaria.

The following investigations and interventions are recommended therefore, at the peripheral levels:

(a) Investigations should be conducted on: the clinical epidemiology of malaria, including clinical and epidemiological characteristics of patients presenting at the various levels of the health-care system; relative numbers of deaths from malaria observed at each level especially 'silent deaths' occurring in the homes; knowledge, attitudes and practices of the population, the health workers and other individuals (such as itinerant drug pedlars) regarding malaria, its risk factors and its treatment.

(b) National malaria policies should be reinforced or established, based on information available on the particular situation of each country. Important points of such policies include guidelines for case management and drug use; criteria for referral to a more central facility; establishment and maintenance of an infrastructure; assurance of a timely supply of drugs to be used at peripheral levels; establishment and maintenance of a health information system including malaria mortality and morbidity among its components.

(c) Populations and health workers in endemic areas should be motivated and educated regarding important aspects of malaria such as prevention, recognition of symptoms, and importance of a rapid and correct treatment.

Malaria health workers at all levels should be provided with clear guidelines on management of malaria. Such guidelines could be provided as simple, standard protocols whose distribution to all workers, especially those involved in direct patient care at the periphery, should be assured. In addition, a simplified version of the WHO's recent publication on severe and complicated malaria (WHO, 1990) would prove useful.

Investigation on the supportive management of severe malaria should include:

(a) Treatment/prevention of hypoglycaemia in severe malaria by the oral administration of dextrose at peripheral levels, where facilities for intravenous perfusion or injections of dextrose do not exist.

(b) Prevention of seizures, especially in African children with cerebral malaria who seem less responsive to phenobarbitone (see chapter by K. Marsh *et al.*). Suggested studies include dose-finding, pharmacokinetic studies to evaluate the effectiveness of intramuscular phenobarbitones, and intragastric phenytoin.

(c) Prevalence of intracranial hypertension in severe malaria and effectiveness of potential preventive/therapeutic measures such as osmotic diuretics.

(d) Treatment of lactic acidosis in severe malaria, using intravenous bicarbonate and dichloroacetate, as well as peritoneal dialysis and haemodialysis.

Recommendations made for investigations on specific management of clinical malaria include the following:

(a) Although parasite clearance times still remain useful, the effective criteria for such trials should be the clinical outcomes of the patients.

(b) Artemisinine derivatives should be evaluated in the treatment of severe malaria. This applies especially to Africa, where the promising results obtained in Asian patients need to be confirmed. Intramuscularly administered derivatives, if efficacious, would prove useful in peripheral health posts where facilities for intravenous drug administration are not available. Similarly, the administration of artemisinine derivatives in suppositories (Arnold *et al.*, 1990) would provide a valuable approach in homes or health posts where injections are not possible.

(c) Sulfadoxine–pyrimethamine, administered intramuscularly, should be investigated. Although this compound offers the advantage of requiring a

single injection, the occurrence of sulfadoxine–pyrimethamine-resistant strains of *Plasmodium falciparum* represents a major handicap.
(d) Preparations counteracting the effect of cytokines should be investigated.

Anaemia and malaria constitute major (and causally linked) sources of morbidity and mortality in the tropics, where safe sources of blood are frequently not available (Greenberg *et al.*, 1988). The health impact of anaemia should be minimized and investigations conducted on:

(a) Criteria for administering blood transfusion in severe anaemia. Such criteria should be based on laboratory biological parameters (such as haemoglobin) as well as functional parameters (such as cardiorespiratory function).
(b) The potential consequences of antimalarial treatments that provide symptomatic cure without parasitological clearance, especially in terms of causing persistent chronic anaemia. This applies particularly to areas where, in spite of chloroquine resistance, national policies continue to recommend chloroquine for the symptomatic treatment of malaria.

Clinical trials should be designed and conducted following rigorous scientific and ethical standards.

A standard randomized controlled format should be adopted whenever possible. Meaningful results should be ensured by enrolling a sufficient number of patients, to be achieved if necessary by using a multicentre format. Such multicentre trials, if well standardized, could profitably include clinical facilities in different countries/continents, thus addressing the issue of epidemiological diversity of clinical malaria and its management. They would also provide a valuable means for transferring expertise and technology in malaria treatment and research.

References

Arnold K, Tran Tinh Hien, Ngyen Tran Chinh, Nguyen Hoan Phu and Pham Phuong Mai (1990) A randomized comparative study of artemisinine (qinghaosu) suppositories and oral quinine in acute falciparum malaria. *Transactions of the Royal Society of Tropical Medicine and Hygiene*, 84, 499–502

Deming, MS, Gayibor A, Murphy K, Jones TS and Karsa T (1989) Home treatment of febrile children with antimalarial drugs in Togo. *Bulletin of the World Health Organization*, 67, 695–700

Greenberg AE, Nguyen-Dinh, P, Mann, JM *et al.* (1988) The association between malaria, blood transfusions, and HIV seropositivity in a pediatric population in Kinshasa, Zaire. *Journal of the American Medical Association*, 259, 545–549

Greenwood, BM, Bradley AK, Greenwood AM *et al.* (1987) Mortality and morbidity from malaria among children in a rural area of The Gambia, West Africa. *Transactions of the Royal Society of Tropical Medicine and Hygiene*, 81, 478–486

WHO (1990) Severe and complicated malaria, 2nd edition. *Transactions of the Royal Society of Tropical Medicine and Hygiene*, 84 (suppl. 2), 1–65

Environmental management in malaria control in India

Vinod P. Sharma

Malaria Research Centre, Delhi, India

Introduction

Every fifth person in India used to suffer from malaria during the pre-DDT era and the loss of human lives was very great. India is basically an agricultural country, with 75–80% of her population dependent on a rural economy. The dream of successful malaria control was almost fulfilled soon after the Second World War by the residual killing action of DDT and its large-scale application in public health.

There had been several examples of successful malaria control by environmental management methods from throughout the world (for example in the USA in Tennessee Valley: Gartrell *et al.*, 1981; in Malaysia: Field and Reid, 1956; in Indonesia: Snellen, 1987; and in India: Covell, 1928; Clyde, 1931; Russell and Knipe, 1942; Rao and Nassiruddin, 1945). However, the spectacular control achieved by DDT overshadowed other approaches and in the euphoria that followed the near-eradication of malaria environmental management methods were almost forgotten. Malaria, however, returned with a vengeance. Today indigenous malaria transmission occurs in the world in a hundred countries, and 83% of the cases reported to WHO annually (excluding the African region) are concentrated in nine countries: Afghanistan, Brazil, China, India, Mexico, Philippines, Sri Lanka, Thailand and Vietnam (WHO, 1990).

The spraying of DDT and other residual insecticides under the National Malaria Eradication Programme (NMEP) had nearly eradicated malaria from India in the early 1960s. This success was followed by a period of focal outbreaks and large-scale resurgence in 1970s, which peaked in 1976 when 6.45 million parasite-positive cases were reported by the NMEP (Sharma and Mehrotra, 1986). Following this resurgence a more realistic approach to malaria control was adopted by the government in 1977 under the modified plan of operation (Pattanayak and Roy, 1980). The 'eradication approach' was scrapped in favour of 'control', to be achieved by emphasizing residual insecticidal spraying in endemic areas with an annual parasite index (API) of two or more and drug distribution to all fever cases. As a result there was a gradual reduction in numbers of reported cases to about 2 million in the early 1980s.

India is spending about US$100 million annually on the control of rural and urban malaria. The targeted populations under DDT, HCH and malathion spray coverage are 220, 122 and 24 million, respectively, but there has been no improvement in the past decade and the number of reported cases has remained at about 2 million annually, 35% of these due to *Plasmodium falciparum* (Sharma, 1990). In spite of spraying, large areas remain endemic, fulminating epidemics occur in areas under the cover of insecticides and spraying has become ineffective. Increasing financial constraints have made the field operations possible only in high transmission areas (API of 10 or 20 or more). Several independent studies in the country have shown that the malaria cases reported by the NMEP at best reflect only the trend and may be the 'tip of the iceberg'.

Environmental management — some considerations

The need for Environmental Management in vector control arose because

(1) Spraying is gradually failing to interrupt transmission.
(2) Spraying of pesticides on a regular basis is hazardous, and contaminates the environment and the food chain.
(3) The high cost of insecticides results in shortages, e.g. in 1983–1989 35% of the malaria budget was spent on insecticides (DDT 75% wettable powder, 11 574 tonnes; HCH 50% wettable powder, 14 505 tonnes; and malathion 25% wettable powder, 12 933 tonnes) and the population coverage was only 47.4%.
(4) There is misuse of insecticides.
(5) There are operational failures.
(6) The social unacceptability results in a high rate of refusals (< 30–40% room coverage is achievable).
(7) Insecticide resistance in vector species necessitates use of replacement insecticides which are costly, hazardous and may push the costs beyond affordable limits.
(8) Spraying has harmful effects on beneficial fauna.
(9) There is a lack of collateral benefits.
(10) Spraying is not effective in stable malaria areas as DDT use has not interrupted transmission after more than a decade of continuous spraying among the 9% of the population who live in hard-core areas, and in areas of unstable malaria quinquennial peaks are encountered even under the cover of insecticides.

Environmental management of vector control has none of the problems connected with insecticides, and long-term control of mosquito breeding is attainable in harmony with nature. The method, if applied properly, has the capacity to eradicate malaria from some areas, and works in areas refractory to spraying. Integration of this strategy with the overall developmental plan for the region can bring holistic development with benefits to society.

Therefore during the VI plan (1980–1985) it became clear that spraying was not the answer to malaria control and the logical solution would be to reduce receptivity and vulnerability by the application of environmental management, biological control, involvement of various sectors of government and eliciting active support and participation of the communities.

Broadly speaking the methods comprise:

(1) environmental management, which includes modification, manipulation and habitat management;
(2) biological control, in which *Gambusia affinis* (gambusia) and *Poecilia reticulata* (guppy) have been used extensively;
(3) early case detection and prompt radical treatment by organizing good surveillance on a weekly basis;
(4) health education to bring awareness and elicit community participation.

Efforts were also made to support interventions by involving the departments of irrigation and forestry, construction agencies, by invoking legislative measures and by encouraging people's participation with incentives in the form of edible fish culture and forestry plantation in waste land (Sharma, 1987). The first project on bioenvironmental control of malaria was launched in 1983 in Kheda district (Gujarat) and extended in phases to 11 more endemic locations in the country. The project has an annual budget the equivalent of US$1.5 million and employs a staff of 425, with 50 scientists and a large workforce. Results of the field studies in some malaria-endemic areas are briefly described in this chapter.

Rural malaria control

Anopheles culicifacies is the primary vector of rural malaria in India. It breeds in a variety of habitats such as ponds, puddles, ditches, rainwater collections, borrow pits, irrigation channels, seepages, ricefields, hoof-prints, etc. The breeding increases enormously and covers vast areas with the onset of the rains and therefore environmental management of vector breeding becomes very difficult. The vector has become resistant to DDT and HCH in almost all parts of the country and to malathion in Gujarat, Maharashtra, Madhya Pradesh and Andhra Pradesh. Basically the vector is zoophilic but it has the capacity to maintain high endemicity to precipitate epidemics and in certain places to maintain persistent malaria transmission. In some areas transmission by *An. fluviatilis* (which prefers human blood and breeds in streams) exceeds that due to *An. culicifacies*. Both vectors transmit *P. vivax* and *P. falciparum*. It is estimated that about 60–70% of malaria cases are generated annually by *An. culicifacies* alone, and 70–80% of NMEP's expenditure is incurred in the control of this vector.

In Kheda district there was an epidemic of malaria before the project was launched and in some villages there were deaths due to malaria. This area was predominantly *P. vivax* but *P. falciparum* cases increased suddenly. Seven villages were selected from one location (population 26 000) and in this population 4040 cases (685 *P. falciparum*) were recorded in 1981 by the malaria department. Work on malaria control was started in 1983 and in 1984 bioenvironmental interventions were intensified and spraying was withdrawn. To improve case detection, surveillance was instituted on a weekly basis instead of at fortnightly intervals. In 1985 the study was extended to cover 14 more villages (population 59 000) and in 1986 the entire Nadiad taluka comprising 100 villages (population 348 000) was covered. In 1987 inclusion of Kapadwanj taluka increasd the population to 686 000 and in 1988 to 695 000.

Analysis of specific breeding sites showed control of *An. stephensi*. Weekly surveys showed that in wells positivity for mosquito breeding was 13–46% in the project area as compared to 69–100% in the control area. When there was breeding in the project area it was generally of low intensity, but some newly positive wells were discovered and in some wells guppies either died or were incompletely effective owing to the presence of debris. The mosquito breeding was more effectively controlled when, late in 1985, expanded polystyrene (EPS) beads were applied in disused wells which are mainly sites of *Culex* breeding (Sharma *et al.*, 1985). Mosquito breeding in ponds and ditches was controlled very effectively by guppies but periodical weeding was necessary. In some village ponds, combined culture of carp and guppies was demonstrated which increased income of Panchayats (village councils) and this money was used in vector control (Gupta *et al.*, 1989). Health education was intensified in the schools and by house-to-house visits, exhibitions were organized, radio talks were given and several films on the field-work were transmitted on television in the regional language. Voluntary labour camps (Shram Dan) were periodically organized to fill up pits, ditches and low-lying areas, and extensive marshy areas were planted with eucalyptus. The impact of the interventions was appreciated at all levels of government and particularly by the communities. There was reduction in *An. culicifacies* densities (Table 1) but this species was not fully eliminated partly owing to the extensive breeding opportunities during the transmission season and possibly as a result of immigration. The study clearly demonstrated successful control of peri- and intra-domestic breeding and control in wells and ponds which was reflected in the reduced adult *An. culicifacies* populations.

Parasitological evaluation of interventions is given in Table 2. In the project villages case detection was better (annual blood examination rate, ABER, was high) and there was reduction in transmission from 1984 to 1986. The annual parasite index (API) and annual falciparum index (AfI) fell from 16 and 3.4 in 1983 to 1.8 and 0.6 in 1986, respectively. In 1987 there was some increase in numbers of malaria cases (API 2.8, AfI 0.7), thought to be due to the fact that the interventions were not as uniform and effective as in previous years because of

Table 1   *An. culicifacies* densities (collection per man hour) during the rainy season (July to September) in the project and control villages

Year	Human dwellings		Mixed human and animal dwellings		Cattle sheds	
	Project area	Control	Project area	Control	Project area	Control
1984	4.12	6.00	8.8	15.30	12.00	27.00
1985	1.37	7.11	2.8	16.77	4.77	19.44
1986	1.70	4.10	2.7	6.00	4.70	5.70

Source: In-depth evaluation report, 1987.

the doubling of the intervention area in one year, and case histories also revealed imported cases (Sharma and Sharma, 1988).

In 1988 there was a sudden increase in cases resulting from water inundation in borrow pits created to extend the canal adjacent to the project areas. Heavy *An. culicifacies* breeding influenced 15–20 villages and an epidemic broke out in that area. Intensive antimalaria operations (spraying and early treatment) reduced transmission in 1989. In comparing the results (see Table 2) it became clear that the trend of transmission in the project and sprayed areas was similar. It should be pointed out that the bioenvironmental strategy was implemented in the post-epidemic period, when there was a declining trend of malaria in the region.

Table 2   Epidemiological indices of malaria in Kheda district

	Project area				Control area (Pop. 3.2 m)		
Year	Pop. (in thousands)	No. cases	API (AfI)	ABER	No. Pf cases	API (AfI)	ABER
1983	26	418 (89)	16 (3.4)	15.4	28247 (1045)	8.8 (0.3)	15.1
1984*	26	141 (64)	5.6 (2.6)	45.8	17754 (670)	5.5 (0.2)	15.2
1985*	59	154 (52)	2.6 (0.9)	34.5	6822 (433)	2.1 (0.14)	14.5
1986*	348	626 (211)	1.8 (0.6)	29.6	7753 (1400)	2.4 (0.43)	18.8
1987*	686	1938 (511)	2.8 (0.7)	29.3	14149 (1729)	4.4 (0.54)	21.6
1988*	695	6265 (3926)	9.0 (5.7)	28.1	20880 (7639)	6.5 (2.4)	20.8
1989	360	1476 (548)	4.1 (1.5)	8.8	12273 (1831)	5.3 (0.6)	9.8

* Bioenvironmental interventions implemented and spraying withdrawn. In other years in the project and control area HCH/malathion and DDT were sprayed.
API = annual parasite index, AfI = annual falciparum index, ABER = annual blood examination rate, Pf = *Plasmodium falciparum*.

In Kheda the main problem was lack of inter-sectoral coordination particularly from the irrigation department. The canal lining was damaged and in general canal maintenance was poor, as revealed by lack of weeding operations and the practice of illegal irrigation. Therefore there was profuse breeding in the canals, tributaries and seepages, etc., the control of which was near impossible without the active support of the irrigation department. One of the most important factors for the success of environmental management in rural malaria control is the inter-sectoral coordination, with the irrigation department made accountable for the proper maintenance of canals.

In 1988 the Gujarat government decided to implement the environmental management strategy through the district infrastructure and general health services. Project resources were diverted to preparatory work related to the transfer of technology to cover the entire Kheda district — a population of 3.5 million and seven urban centres. In direct cost analysis the bioenvironmental strategy was found to be the least expensive of the options considered. Costs per capita of different methods in 1987 were: (a) bioenvironmental control, US$0.29; (b) DDT spray, US$0.36; (c) HCH spray, US$0.38; and (d) malathion spraying, US$1.31. There appeared to be further scope for cost reduction through more research and development of better management and expansion of the area/population coverage under the project so as to reduce overheads (Indepth evaluation report, 1987).

The study was extended to Dadraul Primary Health Centre (PHC) villages of Shahjahanpur district (Uttar Pradesh). In this area seven main rivers and the Sharda canal tributaries provide innumerable mosquito breeding sites. Extensive areas are low lying and waterlogged. Mosquito nuisance was very high and so were the *An. culicifacies* populations. In 1983, a serious epidemic of falciparum malaria took a heavy toll; district authorities recorded 349 deaths due to malaria in Negoyi and Tilhar PHCs (Sharma *et al.*, 1985b). Several focal outbreaks were also reported in Dadraul PHC. Studies showed a high parasite load in the community, and DDT and HCH resistance in *An. culicifacies*.

In May 1986, bioenvironmental interventions were launched in 21 villages, and five adjacent villages were held as controls. Intervention methods were the same as applied in Kheda. In Shahjahanpur *Gambusia* was allowed to multiply in village ponds and wells. In about two years the fish increased in numbers sufficiently to allow the introduction into almost all ponds, ditches and wells all over the district. EPS beads were applied to disused wells. As a result mosquito breeding was greatly reduced and so were the *An. culicifacies* densities, and consequently malaria transmission. The slide positivity rate fell from 70-80% to <5% (Figure 1). An experiment was launched in eight villages to study the impact of *G. affinis* alone on mosquito breeding and adult vector densities. A comparison with control villages (Figure 2) showed that *G. affinis* almost completely eliminates mosquito breeding, but the impact on adult densities was not as pronounced perhaps because of immigration of mosquitoes from outside

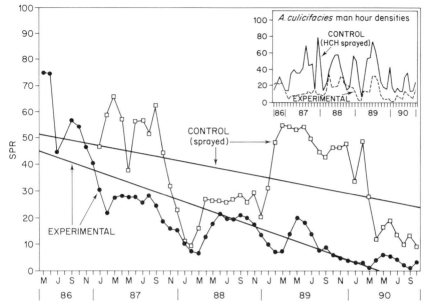

Figure 1 Impact of bio-environmental interventions in Shahjahanpur on the slide positivity rate (SPR) in experimental and control villages (main graph) and *An. culicifacies* densities per man hour (Inset). HCH was sprayed in the control but not the experimental villages. (Source: Dr R.N. Prasad and co-workers Shahjahanpur)

the experimental areas. In this area as well as at other places *Gambusia* is cultured along with carp for human consumption without any harmful effects to either species.

Industrial malaria control

Most of the industrial complexes in India are located in areas with moderate-to-high risk of malaria. At the Bharat Heavy Electricals Ltd (BHEL) plant malaria was responsible for high morbidity (at least every 15th person was afflicted and some repeatedly) with occasional deaths, and there was an increase in the incidence of falciparum malaria. A feasibility study of malaria control by environmental management methods was therefore undertaken. BHEL is spread over 25 km² southwest of Hardwar (Uttar Pradesh), originally with a population of 45 000 (now 65 000) living in seven planned and seven unauthorized colonies. It has excellent medical facilities, with a 180-bed hospital and five dispensaries. Malaria control was based on larviciding, malathion fogging, occasional spraying of hutments and treatment of cases. BHEL staff quarters have screened doors and windows.

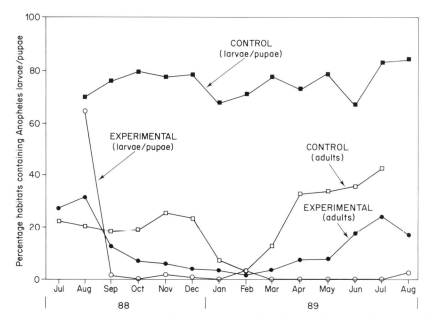

Figure 2 Impact of *Gambusia affinis* on immature (pooled data from wells and ponds) and adult *Anopheles* densities in 8 experimental and 3 control villages in Dadraul PHC district Shahjahanpur (Source: Haq and co-workers, Shahjahanpur)

A survey revealed that the BHEL site had innumerable mosquito breeding sites, some natural but mostly man-made. Mosquito nuisance on the site was high, and as already mentioned there was active malaria transmission, with falciparum malaria showing an alarming increase. Commonly encountered breeding sites were borrow pits, low-lying areas, ponds, ditches, faulty water supply resulting in water stagnation, blocked drains, overhead water tanks, a seasonal river, streams, discarded containers and coolers. To assist in controlling breeding, all potential mosquito breeding sites were mapped. A village 5 km away with a population of 1000 was held for comparison (without any intervention). Project staff carried out vector control, and parasitological examination and treatment were done by hospital staff in collaboration with the project staff.

The main intervention methods consisted of diverting the thermal power fly-ash to fill borrow pits, ditches and low-lying areas. In addition there was canalization of drains and application of EPS beads to sluice valves. Water taps were shifted from low-lying areas to better gradient levels, soakage pits were constructed, and breeding of mosquitoes close to homes was controlled. In marshy areas eucalyptus was planted and many filled-up areas were converted to parks and playgrounds. Environmental interventions were supported by

weekly active surveillance and treatment was given to malaria patients within
24–36 hours of detection of a case.

Pre-intervention vector densities in August 1986 were 11–20 per man hour.
Interventions started in September 1986 and by January 1987 work was in
progress on the entire site. Figure 3 shows the impact of the intervention
measures. Vector densities (*An. culicifacies, An. fluviatilis, An.
stephensi*) were almost completely eliminated except for a small peak (a density per man hour of
about 10) during the rainy season. In the control village densities were very high
and peak density per man hour ranged from 100 to 150. The impact of
intervention was visible in the initial year (1986). In 1987 there was a very sharp
drop in the incidence, suggesting near-interruption of transmission. This drop
was initially suspected to be due to drought, but the following years had good
rainfall and malaria cases have remained at less than 500 per year (Dua *et al.*,
1988). Epidemiological investigations revealed that most cases (up to 60 %) were
imported or contracted outside, and some were relapses, leaving about 20–25 %

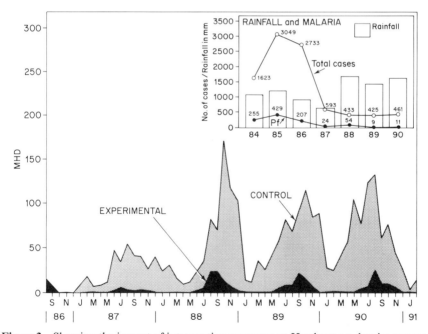

Figure 3   Showing the impact of intervention measures at Hardwar on density per man
hour of vectors (mainly *An. culicifacies* + small populations of *An. fluviatilis* and *An.
stephensi*). Inset shows yearwise incidence of malaria and rainfall. Sudden drop in malaria
cases during 1987 was suspected to be due to drought but malaria cases have continued
to decline even in years of heavy rainfall (Source: V.K. Dua and co-workers, Hardwar)

cases where no history of infection from outside or at an earlier time could be ascertained. Transmission of *P. falciparum* at the site has now been interrupted.

Cost-effectiveness studies at BHEL revealed that direct annual loss due to malaria was estimated to be the equivalent of US$0.47 million and the control cost for the first three years was US$0.2 million and thereafter the maintenance cost US$0.05 million per year.

The study was extended in 1987 to the India Drugs and Pharmaceuticals Ltd (IDPL) site at Rishikesh, an industrial complex about 40 km away from BHEL. On this site malaria was a serious problem and mosquito nuisance was considerable. At the outskirts of the site waste water of the IDPL was discharged into a 5-km² swampy area which was the main site of heavy mosquito breeding. In this area a channel was constructed and waste water was diverted into a drain. Fly-ash was used to fill the borrow pits and low-lying areas and other methods of intervention were essentially the same as applied at BHEL. At the IDPL malaria treatment was based on clinical diagnosis. Table 3 gives data on the annual distribution of antimalarials by the hospital. Soon after the interventions in 1987 there was a major reduction in the use of antimalarials and by 1990 antimalarial distribution was reduced by 92–100%. These studies clearly demonstrated that malaria control by environmental management was feasible, practical and made economic sense, and vector breeding could be controlled even in years of high rainfall, if water ponding was eliminated and good drainage ensured.

Urban malaria control

The government of India launched its Urban Malaria Scheme (UMS) in 1971 in towns with a population of more than 40 000 and showing an API of 2 or more with an ABER of at least 10% (Pattanayak *et al.*, 1981). The scheme was to be implemented in 133 towns in phases, and at present 122 towns are under the UMS. Malaria control is carried out by antilarval methods. Preventive measures such as mosquito proofing of overhead tanks (OHTs) and wells are not

Table 3 Distribution of antimalarials by the IDPL hospital

	1985–86	1986–87	1987–88	1988–89	1989–90	Percentage reduction*
Chloroquine tablets	42300	44000	7100	1100	1300	97
Primaquine tablets	11700	6300	3000	1000	984	92
Metakelfin tablets	6040	8000	4500	2100	307	95
Chloroquine (injection 30 ml)	100	88	40	—	—	100

*During 1989–90 compared with 1985–86 pre-intervention year.

applied, fish are not maintained and legislative measures are not implemented except in Bombay.

Madras was selected for bioenvironmental control as 50–70% of the malaria cases (40–50 thousand) in the whole of Tamil Nadu state come from Madras alone. The intervention strategy adopted was:

(1) mosquito proofing of OHTs;
(2) application of EPS beads and or *Gambusia* in OHTs, wells, cisterns and other stagnant water bodies;
(3) lectures in schools, video shows, discussions and house-to-house visits organized on a routine basis to educate people on the preventive methods against mosquito breeding;
(4) maintenance of a clinic but no active surveillance except some mass blood surveys and epidemiological investigations.

Madras city is divided into 150 corporation divisions with a population of about 40 million. The study was launched in March 1987 in corporation division numbers 86, 87 and 88 and in January 1988 in divisions 53, 54 and 55. The total population in these six corporation divisions is 0.2 million. Anna Nagar (population 35 000) was held as a control. The impact was monitored by entomological indices. Data collected by Madras Corporation through the clinics and hospitals were used in parasitological evaluation. Pre-intervention surveys in divisions 86–88 in November to December 1986 revealed breeding by anopheline mosquitoes in 21.3–30.7% of OHTs, 8.3–28.0% of wells and 14.0% of cisterns. In the pre-intervention survey of divisions 53–55 carried out in November to December 1987, the corresponding figures were 31.2–52.2% for OHTs, 18.3–35.9% for wells and 16.2–18.5% for cisterns.

The impact of interventions on breeding habitats was considerable. Less than 5% of the habitats had evidence of mosquito breeding (mostly early instars were found) whereas in the control area 20–60% of OHTs, wells and cisterns were found supporting mosquito breeding (Figure 4). Collection of *An. stephensi* biting cattle per man hour of collection was very low (1/10 or less) in both groups of experimental divisions as compared with the control areas (see Figure 4).

Parasitological data are given in Table 4. Reduction in the slide positivity rate (SPR) in divisions 86–88 between the pre-intervention year 1986 and 1990 was 62.1% ($p < 0.05$). A reduction of 20% occurred in divisions 53–55 but there was an increase in *P. falciparum* cases of 71.3% in 1990 (from 513 to 879) compared with the previous year.

Epidemiological investigations revealed that (a) the five divisions adjoining the six experimental divisions had high breeding potential and up to 85% OHTs supported breeding, and (b) the experimental areas are important commercially and attract a large labour force and businessmen: 176 (33.7%) of the 522 cases investigated in 1989 were imported.

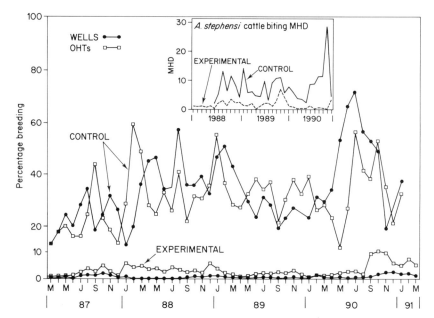

Figure 4   Impact of bioenvironmental interventions on mosquito breeding in overhead water tanks and wells in the corporation divisions 86–88 and 53–55, Madras city. Inset shows the impact on *An. stephensi* adult populations as monitored in the cattlesheds, based on mosquitoes caught biting cattle per man hour of collection between 1800 h and 2000 h. (Source: R.K. Chandrahas and co-workers, Madras)

Table 4   Results of blood smear examination from the experimental areas as recorded by Madras Corporation through passive surveillance

Year	Experimental area	No. of blood smears examined	No. positive (%)		Pf cases	ABER	SPR
1986	86–88	15 895	1041	(6.5)	7	15.90	6.6
1987*	86–88	19 261	978	(5.1)	82	25.20	5.1
1988	86–88	20 367	1199	(5.9)	8	26.52	5.9
1989	86–88	25 380	874	(3.4)	1	27.30	3.4
1990	86–88	15 201	374	(2.5)	1	19.21	3.7
1986	53–55	36 431	5720	(15.7)	716	36.40	15.7
1987	53–55	44 030	6703	(15.2)	992	45.86	15.2
1988**	53–55	43 253	6168	(14.3)	415	45.05	14.3
1989	53–55	48 386	6839	(14.1)	513	39.74	14.1
1990	53–55	43 324	5459	(12.6)	879	56.85	12.6

Intervention started: * March 1987, ** January 1988.
ABER = annual blood examination rate, SPR = slide positivity rate, Pf = *Plasmodium falciparum*.

General conclusions

In reviewing field-work the following points have emerged which may influence the successful implementation of environmental management in malaria control in endemic countries:

(1) Malaria is a local and focal disease involving man, vector, parasite and the environment. Successful implementation of environmental management requires a sound understanding of the transmission dynamics of malaria and the ecosystems involved.

   In most endemic countries, malaria control/eradication programmes have been integrated with general health services under the primary health care approach. This policy has resulted in near-collapse of field operations due to lack of experience in malaria, aggravated by frequent transfers, large numbers of vacancies, uncertain tenure and inertia. As a result malaria incidence and its impact are grossly underestimated, and there is reluctance to accept new approaches.

(2) In contrast to insecticide usage, environmental management reduces the vulnerability of an area to malaria transmission and to areas not responsive to insecticide, and in certain situations environmental management alone may be enough. However, environmental management should not be viewed to the exclusion of other methods such as spraying of insecticides but as complementary to them.

(3) Environmental management in areas of unstable malaria may be successfully applied during the inter-epidemic period, which may be five to seven years or more. This policy will reduce receptivity, costs, insecticide pollution and delay vector resistance to insecticide.

(4) Environmental management does not reduce longevity of vectors, unlike insecticides, and therefore good surveillance is important in curtailing transmission.

(5) Environmental management for vector control requires strong entomological support and leadership. This is weak in most malaria control programmes or at times non-existent. Entomologists do not play a dominant role in decision making at the top level.

(6) Successful environmental management requires a top-down approach with strong political will, social support and sustained inter-sectoral coordination.

(7) Implementation of legislative measures for preventive and corrective action from the very beginning can reduce vector breeding and costs substantially. So far this has been applied to a few urban areas only and there is a need for central legislation.

(8) Environmental management requires some reorganization of health services, taking into consideration the new approaches to vector control, the importance of inter-sectoral coordination, and need for the involvement of

entomologists in decision making. Manpower development, improved research and development, health education and community participation should be strengthened.

(9) In certain areas the initial cost may seem high but environmental management requires a long-term evaluation. Expenditure will be substantially reduced if shared by other sectors. The cost can be further reduced by attacking the vector species only (species sanitation) such as *An. stephensi* in urban areas. Environmental management may also control mosquito nuisance, other disease vectors, produce long-term gains and has the potential for interactions with the industrial and other developmental activities.

(10) Environmental management is less economically viable in areas with low population density. In such areas habitat management, personal protection or bednets may be better approaches to malaria control.

(11) Successful environmental management requires careful planning, execution and monitoring of work, with equal emphasis on maintenance. In most countries budgetary provisions are totally inadequate for maintenance. It may therefore be advisable to stratify the country and prioritize environmental management interventions depending on resource availability.

Acknowledgements

I am grateful to the dedicated project staff working in endemic areas and producing very important and relevant data. In particular I would like to acknowledge the contributions made by the field teams headed by Dr R.C. Sharma (Kheda), Dr R.N. Prasad (Shahjahanpur), Dr V.K. Dua (Hardwar) and Mr R.K. Chandrahas (Madras), whose work constitutes the basis of this chapter. I am also grateful to Dr (Mrs) S.K. Subbarao, Dr (Mrs) Aruna Srivastava and Mrs Poonam Sharma for their help in the preparation of this manuscript.

References

Clyde D (1931) Report on the control of malaria during Sarda Canal construction (1920–1929). *Records of the Malaria Survey of India, 2*, 49–110

Covell G (1928) *Malaria in Bombay.* Government Central Press, Bombay.

Deobhankar PB (1986) Malaria control in Bombay by legislative measures and other non-insecticidal methods of vector control: community participation for disease vector control. Proceedings of the ICMR/WHO workshop to review research results. Malaria Research Centre, Delhi, pp. 101–108

Dua VK, Sharma VP and Sharma SK (1988) Bio-environmental control of malaria in an industrial complex at Hardwar (U.P.), India. *Journal of the American Mosquito Control Association, 4*, 426–430

Field JW and Reid JA (1956) Malaria control in Malaya: an appreciation of the work of Sir Malcolm Watson. *Journal of Tropical Medicine and Hygiene, 59*, 23–27

Gartrell FE, Cooney JC, Chambers GP and Brooks RH (1981) TVA mosquito control 1934–1980: experience and current programme trends and development. *Mosquito News*, *41*, 302–322

Gupta DK, Sharma RC and Sharma VP (1989) Bioenvironmental control of malaria linked with edible fish production in Gujarat. *Indian Journal of Malariology*, *26*, 55–59

In-depth evaluation report (1987) In depth evaluation of the Community Based Integrated Vector Control of Malaria Project in Kheda (Gujarat). MRC, New Delhi, pp. 1–49

Pattanayak S and Roy RG (1980) Malaria in India and the modified plan of operations for its control. *Journal of Communicable Diseases*, *12*, 1–14

Rao BA and Nassiruddin M (1945) Malaria in Irwin Canal area, Mysore state. Part II. *Journal of the Malaria Institute of India*, *6*, 109–128

Russell PF and Knipe FW (1942) A demonstration project in the control of rural malaria by anti-larval measures. *Journal of the Malaria Institute of India*, *4*, 615–631

Sharma VP (1987) Community based malaria control in India. *Parasitology Today*, *3*, 222–226

Sharma VP (1990) The changing scenario of disease vector control in India. Diamond Jubilee commemoration volume: *Glimpses of Science in India*. National Academy of Sciences, Allahabad, Ed WS Srivastava. Malhotra New Delhi, pp. 69–83

Sharma VP and Mehrotra KN (1986) Malaria resurgence in India: a critical study. *Social Science and Medicine*, *22*, 835–845

Sharma RC and Sharma VP (1988) Epidemiological implications of population migration: Part I. Imported malaria in Kheda district, Gujarat. *Indian Journal of Malariology*, *25*, 113–116

Sharma VP and Sharma RC (1989) Community based bioenvironmental control of malaria in Kheda district, Gujarat, India. *Journal of the American Mosquito Control Association*, *5*, 514–521

Sharma RC, Yadav RS and Sharma VP (1985a) Field trials on application of expanded polystyrene (EPS) beads in mosquito control. *Indian Journal of Malariology*, *22*, 107–109

Sharma VP, Chandrahas RK, Nagpal BN and Srivastava PK (1985b) Follow up studies of malaria epidemic in villages of Shahjahanpur district, U.P. *Indian Journal of Malariology*, *22*, 119–121

Snellen WB (1987) Malaria control by engineering measures: pre-World-War-II examples from Indonesia. International Institute for Land Reclamation and Improvement (ILRI), Wageningen, Netherlands, pp. 8–21

WHO (1990) Global estimates for health situation assessment and projections. *WHO/HST/90.2*, 25

WORKSHOP REPORT AND RECOMMENDATIONS
RAPPORTEUR: CHRISTOPHER F. CURTIS

Renewed emphasis should be given to vector control, especially because of the spread of chloroquine resistance. Even when an effective vaccine is available there will be an important place for vector control. Effective methods are already available but there is a need for new tools for vector control and therefore for research in vector biology and vector–parasite relationships.

Residual adulticides

Residual house spraying has been very successful in the past. It has the advantage that adult mosquitoes are at risk every time that they enter a sprayed house and, given reasonably good spray coverage, little chance that any individual will survive long enough for sporozoites to mature in it. Spraying may be essential to control epidemics.

House spraying has the disadvantages that:

(1) many people *perceive* it as dangerous (without scientific justification);
(2) householders often refuse return visits by spray men;
(3) many *Anopheles* populations are resistant to cheaper insecticides;
(4) some replacement compounds are more costly than bioenvironmental control (this may not apply to modern pyrethroids requiring low dosages);
(5) there is frequent misuse of insecticides, e.g. diversion to agricultural usage;
(6) trained spray teams and complex logistics (timely transportation, etc.) are required.

Bioenvironmental control measures

The following are some of the available methods of bioenvironmental control which could be applied by a community, or on a regionally organized basis:

(1) filling of marshy ground (inapplicable to places where *Anopheles* breed in every hoof-print);
(2) planting of water-avid trees to lower the water table in marshy ground;
(3) fish in ponds, ricefields, disused wells, etc.:
    (a) young stages of edible species;
    (b) edible and larvivorous species as a 'package';
(4) management of irrigation:
    (a) prevention of leakage and vegetation growth in canals;
    (b) intermittent irrigation (not universally applicable);
    (c) variation of the level and control of vegetation in impounded water;
(5) floating layers of polystyrene beads against:
    (a) *An. stephensi* in water tanks in urban areas in south Asia;
    (b) nuisance mosquitoes in wells, pits, etc. to enhance the credibility of vector control programmes which often face public protests that, despite much insecticidal spraying, mosquito biting still occurs (usually due to *Culex quinquefasciatus*, which does not respond well to house spraying).

In almost all of the above cases there is an incentive to apply the methods apart from their contribution to malaria control. This incentive may be in the form of land improvement, fuel wood, food fish, saving of irrigation water or reduction of mosquito nuisance.

Apart from existing endemic areas, bioenvironmental control may be appropriate as a precaution against the reintroduction of malaria into areas where it has been eradicated.

Trials of bioenvironmental control

In recent years there has been much talk about bioenvironmental control but relatively little action. It is therefore much to the credit of Dr V.P. Sharma and the teams from the Malaria Research Centre, based in Delhi, that they have gone out into the field to test these methods on an extensive scale. The accurate assessment of to what extent bioenvironmental control really works is so important it is essential that studies are planned in such a way that there are baseline data for the intervention and control areas to indicate how comparable they would have been if the intervention had not been undertaken. However, in none of the cases described by Dr Sharma can one feel fully confident that the intervention and control areas would have had similar mosquito populations and malaria incidence had the intervention not taken place. In only one case are any baseline data given — in most cases single graph lines are shown for the intervention and the control areas and these lines originate after the intervention is already under way. In the case of the Hardwar trial, a village with a population of 1000 was used as the control for a 25-km^2 industrial site; in the Madras trial the graph begins with the month that the intervention started and already shows a large difference between the intervention and control areas, which strongly suggests that they were ecologically different. Thus critical trials of the effectiveness of bioenvironmental control are still needed — they should be replicated in several intervention and several control areas and there should be baseline data for each of these areas.

Problems with bioenvironmental control

(1) As with all larvicidal methods, any larval breeding sites which are missed will yield potentially long-lived, infective, adult mosquitoes and immigrants into small areas under larval control and high survival prospects (thus in some respects bioenvironmental methods are more demanding than house spraying and meticulous searching out of all breeding sites within mosquito flight range of the community which it is intended to protect will be necessary).

(2) When marshy areas are filled, any small pools left would favour certain vector species, such as *An. gambiae*, and could make the situation worse.

(3) Inappropriate drainage and tree planting could be ecologically harmful.

(4) In some countries there is a lack of the necessary skilled manpower to carry out some forms of bioenvironmental control; there are frequent failures of inter-sectoral coordination (e.g. between health and irrigation departments) and, if there are laws against practices which encourage mosquito breeding, they are seldom enforced.

(5) Bioenvironmental methods are inapplicable in areas of low human population density.

Bednets treated with pyrethroids for malaria control

Lu Bao Lin

Institute of Microbiology and Epidemiology, Beijing, People's Republic of China

Introduction

Bednets are widely used against mosquitoes or for other insects in many countries, including China. It is generally assumed that the bednets reduce malaria transmission. However, for various reasons, bednets do not give sufficient protection against mosquito bites. In order to strengthen their protective efficacy impregnation of nets with DDT or other chemicals was suggested but the methods have only recently been put into wide use. During the 1980s the commercial availability of pyrethroids, which are highly insecticidal but with low mammalian toxicity, revived interest in bednets. Trials with bednets treated with these insecticides have since been reported from many countries (WHO, 1989), and the use of treated nets or other materials against malaria vectors has been reviewed by Curtis *et al.* (1989), Rozendaal (1989) and Rozendaal and Curtis (1989).

As the present chapter aims at the practical use of bednets treated with pyrethroids, I shall emphasize the applications of this measure in antimalarial programmes based on experiences in China, and make suggestions for its future use.

Untreated and treated nets

Although the use of bednets is the most popular measure for individual protection against malaria vectors, detailed studies of their efficacy are surprisingly few. Recently Liu *et al.* (1986) carried out a field trial with bednets integrated into a programme of mass drug administration (MDA) from 1980 to 1985 in a township of Jiangsu Province, China. The township, with a population of 26 369, was endemic for vivax malaria transmitted by *Anopheles sinensis*. In 1972–1975 the control measure adopted was simply MDA, including a full course of chloroquine plus primaquine in the non-transmitting season, and chemoprophylaxis with chloroquine (0.3 g) plus primaquine (30 mg) twice a month in the transmitting season for the whole population in addition to case treatment. The annual morbidity rate dropped from 62.5% in 1971 to 0.7% in

1975. However, after the MDA was discontinued the number of malaria cases increased quickly and the incidence reached 18.08% in 1980.

Subsequently, by motivating the villagers to sleep indoors with bednets and reducing infective sources by MDA and case treatment the annual incidence of malaria decreased to 0.45/1000 in 1985. Even after MDA was stopped in 1983 malaria incidence decreased steadily. The conclusion was that the reduction of man–vector contact significantly reduced the transmission rate in the area.

In a small field trial in a Kenyan school Nevill et al. (1988) also reported a reduction of 97.3% in malaria attack rate for children who slept under bednets. However, this highly effective result was obtained under strict supervision. Because of improper use, torn nets and for other reasons bednets usually give only partial protection against mosquito bites. Mosquitoes have been observed to suck blood through a net from the part of the body in contact with it. For example, during a field observation in a town of Jiangsu Province in 1989, of 316 Culex pipiens pallens caught on untreated nets at night and dawn from July to September, as many as 53% were engorged with blood.

Insufficient protection against malarial infection by untreated nets has been reported by Rozendaal et al. (1989), Snow et al. (1988c), Trape et al. (1987) and others. A more detailed analysis of the effectiveness of treated and untreated nets was made in comparative studies in Hainan Island (Li et al., 1988b). The use of untreated nets did not significantly reduce the risk of infection, but the monthly malaria incidence in the group of inhabitants protected with deltamethrin-impregnated nets (1.2/1000) was significantly lower than in those with untreated nets (33.3/1000) or without nets (33.4/1000). It is therefore clear that the effective control of malaria cannot be expected by only routine use of bednets in an endemic area. In order to improve the protective effect of the bednets they should be treated with pyrethroids.

The treatment of bednets in China was initiated during the past decade, showing first the effective reduction of the number of biting mosquitoes on nets impregnated with permethrin (Chao, 1984), and high killing and excito-repellent effects for those treated with deltamethrin (Guangdong Institute of Parasitic Disease Control, 1984; Li and Liang, 1984). Since 1986, treatment of bednets with deltamethrin has been increasingly adopted in antimalarial programmes in many parts of the country.

Operational management of bednet treatment

Up to the present, deltamethrin, either the emulsifiable concentrate (EC) or a wettable powder (WP), is the pyrethroid used most to treat bednets in antimalarial programmes in China; a few field trials have been made with permethrin and alphacypermethrin.

Treatment of nets is carried out by the local health workers with community participation. Impregnation is the method of treatment adopted, with the exception of Sichuan Province, where a spray-on method is practised extensively.

Before impregnation, a quantity of water sufficient to soak each net completely is measured. For ECs the volume to be added to the water to give the desired concentration is calculated. Groups of inhabitants are assembled at appointed localities. Each inhabitant is requested to bring his or her net, washed beforehand, plus a non-absorbing water container such as the washing basin commonly used by the villagers. A health worker in each group measures the quantity of water and puts the amount of EC required into the container. The owner of the net is asked to soak the net by hand rubbing in the diluted solution to obtain uniform distribution of the insecticide over the whole net. The treated net is dried in a shaded place. With good organization the impregnation of more than 20 000 nets can be completed within two days.

For WP the method adopted is similar to that suggested by Snow *et al.* (1988b). The net is dipped into a properly prepared suspension in a large container by the owner and the excess suspension is squeezed out back into the container.

For the spray-on method 2.5 % EC of deltamethrin of 1:100 dilution in water is sprayed on nets with knapsack sprayers at a dosage of 9.6–12 mg/m^2 by local malarial control personnel.

Before spraying silkworms have to be moved out of the room. The malaria control unit of Sichuan Province claimed that the spray-on method had the advantage of simplicity and rapidity in practice and used less insecticide than impregnation. However, impregnation needs no special apparatus and training for practice, and it is easier to control concentrations. No detailed comparison of the effectiveness of the two methods has been made in China.

Bednets treated with deltamethrin

As stated above, the studies on and application of the treated bednets in antimalarial programmes in China were concentrated on the use of deltamethrin. Trials with deltamethrin-impregnated nets were also carried out in Mali (WHO, 1989), Burkina Faso (Carnevale *et al.*, 1988) and India (Jana *et al.*, personal communication).

The results of laboratory studies on the knockdown effect of deltamethrin and permethrin on both cotton and polyester fabrics for three important malaria vectors, *An. anthropophagus*, *An. sinensis* and *An. minimus* are shown in Table 1. On cotton, deltamethrin was much more effective than permethrin. Durability of both pyrethroids was better on cotton than on polyester.

High mortality and long-lasting effects were observed by exposure of *An. anthropophagus* and *An. sinensis* inside the deltamethrin-sprayed nets (9.6 mg/m^2) for 30 minutes (Yang *et al.*, 1990). Average mortality rates of 97.9 % for the former and 95.5 % for the latter were noted after exposure to nets treated

Table 1 Toxic effect (KT50) of deltamethrin and permethrin-treated nets to *An. anthropophagus*, *An. sinensis* and *An. minimus*

			Dosage (mg/m^2)			
Pyrethroid	Mosquito species	Fabric	0.05	0.5	5.0	10.5
Deltamethrin	*An. anthropophagus*	Cotton	23.48	13.68	8.95	5.90
		Polyester	33.44	15.88	14.54	10.44
	An. sinensis	Cotton	40.12	20.04	8.38	6.94
		Polyester	34.26	17.54	10.45	7.94
	An. minimus	Cotton	16.61	13.53		6.55
		Polyester	17.64	9.62		6.99
Permethrin	*An. anthropophagus*	Cotton	52.90	25.71	17.76	14.18
		Polyester	57.72	21.50	11.75	8.95
	An. sinensis	Cotton	60.48	44.25	32.21	23.55
		Polyester	32.47	22.68	8.65	7.66
	An. minimus	Cotton	28.36	17.26	3.87	
		Polyester	14.13	11.90		

Data supplied by Wu Neng.
KT50, minutes of exposure required for 50% of mosquitoes to be knocked down.

1-104 days previously. Bioassays with laboratory-colonized *An. dirus* by similar exposure to deltamethrin-impregnated nets (25 mg/m^2) showed 100% and 98% mortality rates for 306 and 544 days, respectively, after treatment of nets (Li *et al.*, 1988a). It is obvious that such high mortality would not be observed during field applications as mosquitoes would not rest so long on the treated nets because of the excito-repellent effects, but the laboratory results showed clearly the high toxicity of treated nets to mosquitoes making contact with them.

An experimental hut study was carried out in Guangzhou, Guangdong Province, with the use of a penned buffalo or ox as a bait in a closed or semi-closed large net impregnated with deltamethrin (25 mg/m^2), and an untreated net in another hut as control (Li *et al.*, 1988a). High mortality rates of 89.1-99.7% for completely closed nets and 76.3-84.7% for semi-closed nets 755 days after insecticide treatment were observed among *An. sinensis* that entered the huts. A similar experimental hut study was performed in a rice cultivation area of Hanjiang, Jiangsu Province. A mortality rate of 50.5-90.5% for completely closed nets impregnated with 20 mg/m^2 deltamethrin was also noted for *An. sinensis* exposed to nets treated 41 days before (Xu Rongman *et al.*, 1989a).

Both studies showed a reduction of blood sucking and a notable excito-repellency among mosquitoes in contact with treated nets.

Associated pilot field trials were carried out in Guangdong and Sichuan Provinces, with encouraging results. Therefore deltamethrin-treated bednets

Table 2 Number of bednets treated with deltamethrin in antimalarial programmes in China[a] (1986-1988)

Province	Year	Number of nets treated	% nets treated	Population protected	Dosage (mg/m^2)
Hainan	1986	3 748	86.3	9 426	25
	1987	34 109	85.5	71 716	25
	1988	9 870	87.1	21 150	25
Guangdong	1986	185 131	83.6–91.2	269 068	15
	1987	216 725		302 200	15
	1988	201 080		279 548	15
Henan	1986	6 890	94.5	19 311	15
	1987	9 817	95.3	24 714	15
	1988	56 861	95.4		15
Jiangsu	1986	12 799	93.1	22 688	15
	1987	21 435	95.3	39 001	15
	1988	139 504	95.4		15
Sichuan	1986	18 837	96.9	30 304	9.6
	1987	1 489 929	96.1	2 229 082	12
	1988	2 259 286	96.7	3 852 644	12
Total	1986	227 405		350 957	
	1987	1 772 015		2 666 713	
	1988	2 666 601			

[a] Small-scale trials in Yunnan, Guangxi and other provinces are not included.

were extensively adopted into antimalarial programmes against *An. anthropophagus* and *An. sinensis* or *An. dirus* and the number of nets thus treated increased yearly and reached more than 2.6 million in five provinces in 1988 (Table 2).

Effectiveness against *An. anthropophagus* and *An. sinensis*

An. anthropophagus and *An. sinensis* are important vectors of malaria and Brugian filariasis in China. They are sibling species belonging to the *An. hyrcanus* group. *An. sinensis* is the most common and widely distributed anopheline mosquito, covering a vast area south of latitude 45° N and east of longitude 95° E. Though it is mainly zoophilic it plays an important role in the maintenance of the low endemicity malaria in the plains of China (Lu, 1982).

By contrast, *An. anthropophagus* is an anthropophilic and endophilic species. It occurs in the area between 21° and 34° N and is patchy in distribution. As these two species coexist in most of the control areas mentioned below, the good results obtained with deltamethrin or permethrin-treated nets in antimalarial programmes might be more attributed to their impact on *An. anthropophagus*.

As a rule the use of bednets treated with deltamethrin had marked effects on both vectors and malaria infection. For example, in 1985–1987, Li *et al.* (1988c, 1989) carried out field trials of malaria control using deltamethrin-impregnated nets (15 mg/m^2) in Buji District of Baoan County, Guangdong Province. It is a vivax endemic area with a population of 4450. The first impregnation was in June 1985 and the second in April 1986. During the period the number of mosquitoes caught between 22:00 and 23:00 hours on 20 nets was reduced by 93.8 % and the outdoor collection (human bait in an untreated net for 1 hour) by 52.5 %. A comparison of the treated and control areas demonstrated a decrease of 90 % for indoor catches of both species. In the outdoor catches *An. anthropophagus* decreased by 80 % and *An. sinensis* by 36 %.

The malaria incidence also decreased significantly after impregnation, as shown in Figure 1. During July to December 1985 the average monthly incidence was 4.6/1000, as compared with 11.6/1000 during the corresponding period in 1984, with a decrease of 60.4 %. After the second treatment in 1986 the incidence further decreased to 0.85/1000, i.e. a reduction of 81.5 %. In 1987 the average monthly incidence was only 0.3/1000 (Li *et al.*, 1989).

In April 1986 and 1987 the treatment was extended to the whole of Buji District, with a population of 40 000. The average monthly incidence recorded (April to December) was 0.54/1000 and 0.17/1000, a decrease of 64.7 % and 89 %, respectively, as compared with the same period of the previous year.

Similar results were obtained in a field trial in Yuyi County, Jiangsu Province in 1986–1987. The area was endemic for vivax malaria, but with sporadic cases

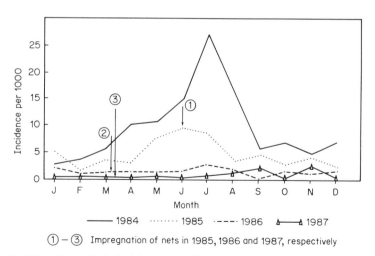

① – ③ Impregnation of nets in 1985, 1986 and 1987, respectively

Figure 1   Monthly malaria incidence of Buji District before and after impregnation of bednets with deltamethrin, 1985–1987 (after Li *et al.*, 1988c)

of falciparum infections. Deltamethrin ($15 \, \text{mg/m}^2$) was used for impregnation of nets in a village with a population of 22 688, covering 93.1 % of 13 725 nets in June. After treatment the number of mosquitoes resting on nets was greatly reduced, with a reduction of 71.2% to 100% from July to October, in comparison with those of the control village. The malaria cases in the treated village from July to December were reduced by 87.5% in comparison with the similar period of 1985 (Table 3) (Lu, 1988). In 1987 the treatment was continued in this village and the annual malaria incidence dropped from 13.5/1000 in 1985 to 1.0/1000 in 1987.

In 1986 bednets in four villages with a population of 30 324 in Yibin County, Sichuan Province, were sprayed with deltamethrin ($9.6 \, \text{mg/m}^2$) (Yang et al., 1990). After treatment the numbers of An. anthropophagus and An. sinensis caught inside the nets were greatly reduced, with an average reduction of 98.8% and 94.3%, respectively. At the same time the outdoor biting rates were reduced by 98.7% for An. anthropophagus and 90% for An. sinensis. A significant lowering of parous rates in both species was also noted.

In the treated villages malaria incidence from July 1986 to May 1987 was reduced by 94.4% in comparison with the corresponding period in the previous year. The parasite rate in school children declined from 4.0% to 0.9%, with a reduction of 80% after treatment.

In the large-scale applications of the method in 1987–1988 (Table 2) the malaria incidence was reduced from 129.2/1000 to 63.9/1000 and 31.2/1000, respectively, with a reduction rate of 50.5% in 1987 and a further reduction of 51.2% obtained in 1988. In 1988 the parasite rates in children were also reduced from 2.2% to 0.78%, a reduction of 64.5%, while a reduction of only 8.7% was found in the control area (Chen et al., 1990).

Effectiveness against *An. dirus*

An. dirus is an important vector in the jungle and hilly regions in Hainan Island. Owing to its strong exophilic behaviour the conventional residual sprays with DDT or other insecticides were not effective for its control.

In 1986 and 1987 Li et al. (1988b) carried out a field trial in a village in Wanning County which was an endemic area for *Plasmodium falciparum* and *P. vivax* malaria in spite of DDT residual spraying. The treated area had a population of 6407, with 3095 nets, and 92% of them were impregnated with deltamethrin (EC $25 \, \text{mg/m}^2$) in April of 1986 and 1987. At the same time deltamethrin was sprayed on the eaves of houses, though subsequent studies suggested that this measure had little effect and it was not repeated in 1987. After treatment, the number of *An. dirus* caught inside the rooms and the biting rates inside and outside houses were all greatly reduced; the malaria incidence was also reduced by 76.7% from 5.87/1000 in 1985 down to 1.66/1000 and 1.35/1000 in 1986 and 1987, respectively (Figure 2). In the control area the corresponding

Table 3 Effectiveness of DDT sprays and deltamethrin and permethrin-impregnated bednets for malarial control in Yuyi County, Jiangsu Province, 1986

Village	Treatment	Malaria incidence, July–December 1985			Malaria incidence, 1986			
		Population	Number of cases	Incidence per 1000	Population	Number of cases	Incidence per 1000	Reduction (%)
1	DDT spray	18 022	75	4.2	17 956	28	1.6	61.90[b]
2	DDT spray	15 244	67	4.4	15 185	53	3.5	20.45
3	DDT spray	16 423	111	6.3	16 369	43	2.6	61.76[b]
4	DDT spray	16 499	37	2.2	16 472	18	1.1	50.00[c]
5	DDT spray	26 739	234	8.8	27 030	19	0.7	92.50[b]
6	DDT spray	16 744	117	7.0	16 796	17	1.0	85.71[c]
7	Deltamethrin[a]	22 600	236	10.4	22 688	30	1.3	87.50[b]
8	Permethrin[a]	27 191	257	9.5	22 993	35	1.3	86.32[b]
9	Control	15 045	32	2.1	15 898	20	1.2	42.86

Adapted from Lu (1988).
[a] Impregnating bednets.
[b] Highly significant statistically ($p < 0.05$).
[c] Significant statistically.

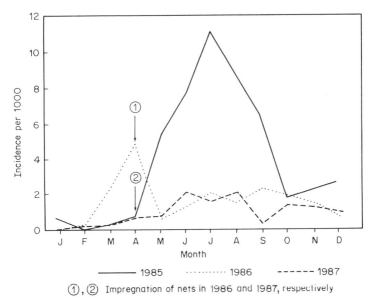

Figure 2 Monthly malaria incidence before and after impregnation of bednets with deltamethrin in Wanning, 1986–1987 (after Li *et al.*, 1988b)

figures were 1.75/1000, 2.45/1000 and 6.19/1000, respectively. Furthermore before treatment 68% of the infections was due to *P. falciparum* but in 1987 all cases were due to *P. vivax*.

The above results of applications of deltamethrin-treated nets invariably showed a reduction in the number of mosquitoes on the nets, and consequently reduction in malaria prevalence by 50% at least. This conclusion is very similar to that in Burkina Faso (Carnevale *et al.*, 1988), where a reduction of 59% was obtained by impregnating nets with deltamethrin.

Bednets treated with permethrin

Permethrin was recommended for use on bednets by a WHO Expert Committee on Vector Biology and Control. It was commonly used for this purpose in many countries other than China. Laboratory and experimental hut studies and field trials on permethrin showed that it shared many features with deltamethrin, such as excito-repellent and toxic effects and reduction in blood feeding and vector density. In addition deterrent and airborne effects were observed in some cases.

Varying results for the effects on malaria were reported from different areas (Rozendaal, 1989) mainly because of differences in malaria endemicity, the proportion of nets treated, the dosage of permethrin used, the habits of the people, and the practical use and handling of nets. However, in most cases reduction of transmission rates was usually obtained and significant reductions in malaria morbidity and/or parasite rates have been reported from The Gambia (Snow et al., 1988a), Papua New Guinea, the Solomon Islands and Vietnam (WHO, 1989).

Permethrin-treated nets had a high knockdown effect, as shown on the three Chinese vectors mentioned above (Table 1). It is considerably more effective on polyester and on nylon (Hossain et al., 1989) than on cotton. High mortality, up to 100%, was observed by exposure of An. sinensis for 1 hour to nets treated (500 mg/m²) 19 weeks previously (Xu et al., 1988). High mortality was also reported for An. balabacensis (Hii et al., 1989), An. culicifacies (Jambulingam et al., 1989), An. maculatus (Loong et al., 1985) and other anophelines by similar exposure.

In the experimental hut studies in Hanjiang, a notable excito-repellent effect was evident from the early departure of An. sinensis (Xu Rongman et al., 1989b), but high mortality of entering mosquitoes was observed only within a week after nets were treated. Some indications of deterrent and airborne effects were noted, but the results were inconclusive.

In the Yuyi field trials mentioned above a parallel study on permethrin-impregnated nets was also conducted in a village with a population of 26 026. Of 13 486 nets in the village, 82.2% were impregnated with permethrin (200 mg/m²). The results showed that their effects on mosquitoes and malaria incidence were comparable to those of deltamethrin-treated nets (Table 3). The number of mosquitoes resting on treated nets at night was reduced by 73.6-100% at periods 5-105 days after treatment (Nie et al., 1989) and malaria incidence was reduced by 85.7% in comparison with that of the similar period in 1985. The annual morbidity rate in the treated villages dropped from 13.8/1000 in 1985 to 0.3/1000 after repeated treatment in 1987 (Nie et al., 1989b).

During these trials indoor residual spraying with DDT was done in six villages of the county, with a combined population of 109 701. An overall reduction of 72.4% (20.5-92.5%) of malaria incidence was noted. The results indicate that the effectiveness of treating bednets with both pyrethroids is comparable to, if not better than, the residual sprays against malaria transmitted by An. anthropophagus and An. sinensis.

A field trial of permethrin-impregnated nets against An. dirus is currently being carried out in Hainan.

From the above results we conclude that the treatment of nets with deltamethrin and permethrin is effective for malaria control in China. However, it has to be pointed out that in all the endemic areas a routine control measure with a course of antirelapse chemotherapy (1.2 g chloroquine for three days and 180 mg primaquine for eight days) is given to persons with a malaria history in the previous year and to the new patients in addition to case treatment.

Safety of pyrethroid-treated nets and cost-effectiveness

All pyrethroids mentioned above have LD50 in rats of more than 2000 mg/kg. They are considered by the WHO as moderately hazardous. Rats exposed to deltamethrin at a dosage of 1500 mg/m^2 for 10 hours daily for 90 days showed no significant difference in psychological, haematological, biochemical and pathological indices from the control group (Lin *et al.*, 1988). The results indicate that the dosage of 15–25 mg/m^2 used for net treatment is probably safe for human beings.

No side-effects were observed in people sleeping under treated nets in the large-scale trials of treated nets in China, Burkina Faso (Carnevale *et al.*, 1988) and other areas.

Furthermore, in China bednets were impregnated in large numbers without the use of gloves as each person impregnated only his or her own net. Apart from some tingling sensation in the skin, no other side-effects have been reported. However, gloves are indispensable for those impregnating many nets.

The cost of treatment with deltamethrin varied from about US$0.05 in Sichuan Province to US$0.10 per capita per year in Jiangsu Province. It was estimated to be about half to one-quarter of the cost of DDT residual sprays and is about half the cost of permethrin treatment in Jiangsu Province in 1986.

Discussion and conclusion

Owing to differences in the socioeconomic conditions, human habits, attitude towards the use of bednets, bionomics of vectors, degree of malaria endemicity and actual practice of control measures it is difficult to generalize about the effectiveness of bednets, particularly those treated with pyrethroids in anti-malarial programmes. However, through the studies made in China and other areas the following points may be noted:

(1) Routine use of untreated bednets is not sufficient to protect against mosquito bites in most cases. The use of bednets can exert an effective impact on malaria infection only under strict supervision, as when linked with MDA.

(2) The protection by the nets can be greatly strengthened by treatment with deltamethrin or permethrin, through their killing and excito-repellent effects. Thus, the number of mosquitoes resting on nets is greatly reduced and consequently their blood sucking. The mosquitoes penetrating into the nets by various means can also be killed by the toxic effect of pyrethroids. In some cases reduction in indoor density and outdoor biting rate of vectors in the treated area is obtained.

(3) The successful application of deltamethrin or permethrin-treated nets in antimalarial programmes in China further demonstrated the effectiveness of

their mass use in low or moderate endemic areas. The experience gained in China is as follows:

(a) The use of treated nets was integrated with the reduction of source of infection by strict antirelapse and case treatment. Recently B.M. Greenwood *et al.* (personal communication) have also demonstrated in The Gambia that better control results were obtained by combining chemoprophylaxis with use of permethrin-treated nets.

(b) The established Chinese tradition of using bednets greatly facilitates the treatment of nets in antimalarial programmes. The percentage of people sleeping under treated nets should be over 60 % of the whole population in the malaria control area in order to obtain effective results.

(c) A good organization is important for the implementation of the treatment. The desired dosages are 15–25 mg/m² for deltamethrin and 200–500 mg/m² for permethrin. One treatment is given each year in China. The inhabitants are asked not to wash their treated nets during the transmission season.

(4) Although the method is effective against both endophilic and exophilic vectors, it is naturally more efficient in the former species. The deltamethrin-treated nets give a higher mortality, but the permethrin-treated nets have stronger excito-repellent effects after contact. However, at present it is hard to judge their relative effectiveness in practical application for malaria control.

(5) In comparison with residual sprays of DDT or other insecticides the use of treated nets has the advantages of better rationale as a control method, simplicity and convenience in application, suitability for primary health care programmes with community participation, reduction in numbers of other nuisance arthropods at the same time, good acceptability by the residents and finally the high cost-effectiveness. In China more and more DDT spray projects have been replaced by treatment of bednets with deltamethrin.

(6) The technical improvements of treatment and problems in the future use have been fully discussed by Rozendaal (1989), Rozendaal and Curtis (1989) and in the report of the WHO (1989). In order to elaborate this promising weapon against malaria some basic studies are particularly important, such as the comparative evaluation of different pyrethroids and their formulations, and the use of available mixtures of deltamethrin or permethrin with other insecticides for impregnation of bednets to prevent or to delay the occurrence of resistance.

Acknowledgement

The writer wishes to thank Professor Jiang Yutu for reading the manuscript and making suggestions. Thanks are also due to Drs B.M. Greenwood, Chen Huailu, Li Mingxin and Wu Neng for providing unpublished papers for reference.

References

Carnevale P, Robert V, Boudin C, Helna J-A, Pazart L, Gazin P, Richard A and Mouchet J (1988) La lutte contre le paludisme par des moustiquaires impregnées de pyrethrinoides au Burkina Faso. *Bulletin de la Société de Pathologie Exotique*, *81*, 832–846

Chao Xuzhong (1984) Field trials of bednets impregnated with permethrin for control of mosquitoes. *Chinese Journal of Preventative Medicine*, *1*, 89 (in Chinese)

Chen Huailu, Liu Chongyi, Kang Wanmin *et al.* (1990) The use of mosquito nets sprayed with deltamethrin in malaria control in Sichuan Province. *Chinese Journal of Parasitic Disease Control*, *3*, 21–23 (in Chinese)

Curtis CF, Lines JD, Carnevale P *et al.* (1990) Impregnated bednets and curtains against malaria mosquitoes. In: Curtis CF (ed.) *Appropriate Technology for Vector Control*. CRC Press, Florida, pp. 5–45

Guangdong Institute of Parasitic Disease Control (1984) Studies on the control of *Anopheles sinensis* and *Anopheles dirus* by bednets impregnated with deltamethrin. *Annals of the Society of Parasitology, Guangdong Province*, *7*, 180–183 (in Chinese)

Hii J, Vun YS, Chin KF *et al.* (1987) The influence of permethrin-impregnated bednets and mass drug administration on the incidence of *Plasmodium falciparum* malaria in children in Sabah, Malaysia. *Medical and Veterinary Entomology*, *1*, 397–409

Hossain MI and Curtis CF (1989) Permethrin impregnated bednets: behavioural and killing effects on mosquitoes. *Medical and Veterinary Entomology*, *3*, 367 76

Hossain MI, Curtis CF and Heekin JP (1989) Assays of permethrin-impregnated fabrics and bioassays with mosquitoes (Diptera: Culicidae). *Bulletin of Entomological Research*, *79*, 299–308

Jambulingam P, Gunasekharan K, Sabu SS, Hota PK, Tyagi BK and Kalyanasundaram (1989) Effect of permethrin impregnated bednets in reducing population of malaria vector *Anopheles culicifacies* in a tribal village of Orissa state (India). *Indian Journal of Medical Research*, *89*, 48–51

Li Mingxin and Liang Zetang (1984) Experiments on the toxic effect of deltamethrin on *Anopheles dirus*. *Annals of the Society of Parasitology, Guangdong Province*, *7*, 184–186 (in Chinese)

Li Zizi, Xu Jinjiang, Li Bangquan, Zu Taihua and Li Mingxin (1988a) Mosquito nets impregnated with deltamethrin against malaria vector in China. In: The studies of bednets impregnated with deltamethrin for the control of vectors and malaria. *Symposium Proceedings, Guangdong Institute of Parasite and Disease Control*, 16–22

Li Zuzi, Zhang Mancheng, Shen Meiwu and Zhang Longfu (1988b) Field trials of deltamethrin impregnated bednets for the control of *Anopheles dirus* transmitted malaria in Hainan Island. In: The studies of bednets impregnated with deltamethrin for control of vectors and malaria. *Symposium Proceedings, Guangdong Institute of Parasite and Disease Control*, 35–49

Li Zuzi, Zhang Mancheng, Wu Yuguang *et al.* (1988c) A 3 year field trial of deltamethrin impregnated bednets for the control of malaria transmitted by *Anopheles sinensis* and *Anopheles anthropophagus*. In: The studies of bednets impregnated with deltamethrin for control of vectors and malaria. *Symposium Proceedings, Guangdong Institute of Parasite and Disease Control*, 24–34

Li Zizi, Zhang Mancheng, Wu Yuguang, Zhong Binglin, Lin Guangyu and Huang Hui (1989) Trial of deltamethrin impregnated bednets for the control of malaria transmitted by *Anopheles sinensis* and *Anopheles anthropophagus*. *American Journal of Tropical Medicine and Hygiene*, *40*, 356–359

Lin Jinyan, Liang Xuemei, Xu Hongjian, Xu Yaru and Chen Guanghua (1988) Simulation toxicity of bednet impregnated with deltamethrin to mammals. In: The studies of bednets impregnated with deltamethrin for control of vectors and malaria. *Symposium Proceedings, Guangdong Institute of Parasite and Disease Control*, 23

Liu Yinlong, Wu Kaishen, Jia Jiaxiang *et al.* (1986) Integrated approach in malaria control including environmental management to reduce man-mosquito contact and reduction of infection source in Huanghuai Plain. *Journal of Parasitology and Parasitic Diseases, 4,* 246–250 (in Chinese)

Loong KP, Naidu S, Thevasagayam ES and Cheong WH (1985) Evaluation of the effectiveness of permethrin and DDT-impregnated bednets against *Anopheles maculatus. Southeast Asia Journal of Tropical Medicine and Public Health, 4,* 544–549

Lu Baolin (1982) The malaria vectors and their control in China. *Chinese Journal of Epidemiology, 3,* 379–338 (in Chinese)

Lu Baolin (1988) The application of deltamethrin treated mosquito nets in anti-malarial programmes in China. In: The studies of bednets impregnated with deltamethrin for control of vectors and malaria. *Symposium Proceedings, Guangdong Institute of Parasite and Disease Control,* 50–56

Nevill CC, Watkins WM, Carter Y and Munafu CG (1988) Comparison of mosquito net, proguanil hydrochloride, and placebo to prevent malaria. *British Medical Journal, 297,* 401–403

Nic Zhaohong, Sun Jun, Chen Zhilong *et al.* (1989a) Application of pyrethroid-impregnated mosquito nets in malaria control. *Bulletin of the Academy of Military and Medical Science, 13,* 39–42 (in Chinese, with English summary)

Nie Zhaohong, Sun Jun, Chen Zhilong, Sun Yucheng, Zhang Yinkuo and Lu Baolin (1989b) Malaria control with deltamethrin impregnated bednets. (1986) *Chinese Journal of Public Health, 8,* 36 (in Chinese)

Rozendaal JA (1989) Impregnated mosquito nets and curtains for self-protection and vector control. *Tropical Diseases Bulletin, 86* (July), R1–41

Rozendaal JA and Curtis CF (1989) Recent research on impregnated mosquito nets. *Journal of the American Mosquito Control Association, 5,* 500–507

Rozendaal JA, Voorham J, Van Hoof JPM and Oostburg BFJ (1989) Efficacy of mosquito nets treated with permethrin in Suriname. *Medical and Veterinary Entomology, 3,* 53–65

Snow RW, Lindsay SW, Hayes RJ and Greenwood BM (1988a) Permethrin treated bednets (mosquito nets) prevent malaria in Gambian children. *Transactions of the Royal Society of Tropical Medicine and Hygiene, 82,* 838–842

Snow RW, Philips A, Lindsay SW and Greenwood BM (1988b) How best to treat bednets with insecticides in the field. *Transactions of the Royal Society of Tropical Medicine and Hygiene, 82,* 647

Snow RW, Rowan KM, Lindsay SW and Greenwood BM (1988c) A trial of bednets (mosquito nets) as a malaria control strategy in a rural area of The Gambia, West Africa. *Transactions of the Royal Society of Tropical Medicine and Hygiene, 82,* 212–215

Trape JF, Zoulani A and Quinet MC (1987) Assessment of the incidence and prevalence of clinical malaria in semi-immune children exposed in intense and perennial transmission. *American Journal of Epidemiology, 126,* 192–201

WHO (1989) The use of impregnated bednets and other materials for vector-borne disease control. *WHO Document WHO/VBC/89.981,* 45 pp

Xu Jinjiang, Zao Meiluan, Luo Xinfu *et al.* (1988) Evaluation of permethrin-impregnated mosquito-nets against mosquitoes in China. *Medical and Veterinary Entomology, 2,* 247–251

Xu Rongman, Lu Baolin, Zie Zhaohong *et al.* (1989a) Experimental hut studies on the effect of deltamethrin-impregnated nets on mosquitoes. *Journal of Preventive Medicine, 7,* 140–145 (in Chinese)

Xu Rongman, Lu Baolin, Chen Xueliang *et al.* (1989b) Experimental hut studies on the

effect of bednets impregnated with permethrin on mosquitoes. *Bulletin of the Academy of Military and Medical Science, 13,* 435–441 (in Chinese with English summary)
Yang Juiping, Liu Guihua, Yang Xingyu *et al.* (1990) Mosquito-net spraying with deltamethrin for malaria control. *Chinese Journal of Parasitology and Parasitic Diseases,* 18–20 (in Chinese, with English summary)

WORKSHOP REPORT AND RECOMMENDATIONS
RAPPORTEUR: PIERRE CARNEVALE

The work in China and elsewhere shows that bednets or curtains impregnated with pyrethroid insecticide provide a valuable tool for vector control that can be applied by a primary health care (PHC) system in which the community participate fully. Untreated bednets are not sufficient to protect people against malaria. Properly used impregnated nets should reduce not only man–vector contact but also transmission of malaria by reducing the population of infective mosquitoes.

Further data are needed on efficacy and feasibility of application of impregnated fabrics.

Efficacy depends on:

(1) active ingredient (to kill and/or to repel mosquitoes);
(2) formulation;
(3) concentration;
(4) resistance/susceptibility of the target population;
(5) nature of the fabric (nylon, cotton, etc.);
(6) application method (dipping/spraying);
(7) persistence of the insecticidal effect in relation to local washing practices of nets;
(8) large-scale use to achieve a 'mass effect';
(9) integration with other methods against vectors and/or parasites.

Efficacy can be evaluated by study of:

(1) entomology;
(2) clinical and parasitological parameters (these depend on the species of parasite, the presence or absence of mass drug administration, local epidemiology);
(3) mortality.

The evaluation methods applied depend on the objectives of the trial.

Feasibility and sustainability of application depend on:

(1) current behaviour of the population in relation to mosquitoes (KAP surveys);
(2) acceptability of nets to the local population and how this could be enhanced;
(3) whether nets are used only against seasonal nuisance mosquitoes;
(4) time and place of biting of the local vector population;
(5) affordability of nets and insecticides (removal of taxation would be helpful);
(6) perception of side-effects of impregnated nets;
(7) existence of an adequate PHC system or other national organizations;
(8) availability of bednets and insecticides of appropriate quality, type and price;
(9) availability of alternative, and possibly more appropriate, types of fabric;
(10) political and social will.

There is a great diversity of epidemiological and sociological situations in malarious areas and we must take these variations into account.

Because of the urgency of the malaria situation, vector control must be carried out by whatever means seems best in the circumstances.

Malaria chemoprophylaxis in endemic regions

Brian M. Greenwood

Medical Research Council Laboratories, Banjul, The Gambia

Introduction

Until relatively recently, the west coast of Africa was notorious as the 'white man's grave'. This reputation was well deserved for mortality among European visitors to West Africa was extremely high. None of the 40 Europeans on Mungo Park's second expedition to the Niger in 1805 survived and mortality on subsequent expeditions to West Africa was extremely high (Ransford, 1983). Missionaries did little better; 60% of the missionaries sent to West Africa by the Church Missionary Society between 1804 and 1825 died. Mortality was also very high among sailors who called at West African ports such as Bathurst (Banjul). Although some of these deaths were probably due to yellow fever and to cholera, there is little doubt that many were caused by malaria.

During the past 10–20 years this situation has changed beyond all recognition. Several hundred thousand tourists visit tropical Africa each year, including many to previously notoriously unhealthy spots such as The Gambia. Although a small proportion of tourists do contract malaria the vast majority enjoy a medically uneventful holiday. How has this dramatic change been brought about? Fifty years ago visitors to Africa made strenuous efforts to protect themselves against mosquito bites through the use of house screening, nets and protective clothes. These measures have now been largely abandoned and tourists expose themselves frequently to the bite of malaria vectors. Thus, there can be little doubt that the main factor that has turned some areas from death traps into tourist resorts has been the advent of safe and effective chemoprophylaxis.

If chemoprophylaxis has been so successful in protecting visitors to highly endemic malaria areas why has this measure not been used widely to protect the local population who are also at risk? There are a number of genuine scientific concerns about the use of chemoprophylaxis in the population of endemic areas which are reviewed later in this chapter. However, it is difficult to escape from the conclusion that the failure to consider prophylaxis as a possible malaria control measure for the local population of endemic areas has been due in part to a hangover from an earlier period when strategies for health care were directed towards the needs of the elite.

During the past few years there has been some change in this attitude and, in this chapter, I shall review the results of several studies which have shown that chemoprophylaxis can benefit the resident population of endemic areas. Some of the drawbacks to this form of malaria control will be considered also; I shall not consider prophylaxis for short-term visitors to endemic areas.

Objectives of chemoprophylaxis for the resident population of endemic areas

When effective synthetic malaria chemoprophylaxis agents, such as pyrimethamine, first became available it was hoped that malaria transmission could be broken in some endemic areas by treatment of the whole population with these drugs. Thus, large-scale trials of mass drug treatment were undertaken, sometimes combined with vector control. Although drug treatment was effective initially at lowering parasite and spleen rates, these rates soon returned to their previous levels once drug administration was stopped (Cavalie and Mouchet, 1962; Escudie et al., 1962). Thus, few people now advocate mass drug treatment as a malaria control measure except under unusual circumstances, for example during an epidemic in an area of usually low transmission. However, mass drug administration was undertaken on a national scale in Nicaragua in 1981, when about 70% of the population were treated with chloroquine and primaquine; this achieved a reduction in the incidence of *Plasmodium falciparum* malaria for a period of about seven months (Garfield and Vermund, 1983). Nevertheless, it is now generally accepted that if chemoprophylaxis is to be used in the population of endemic areas it should not be given to the whole population but should be targeted at the groups most at risk.

In areas where malaria is endemic the major health impact of the infection is on young children, among whom it may cause death from anaemia or from cerebral malaria, and among pregnant women, especially primigravidae, in whom it may cause severe anaemia and placental damage leading to low birth weight. In some endemic areas, for example Thailand and Brazil, migrants of all ages from an area of the country with a low prevalence of malaria to one of high endemicity may also be at special risk. It is these groups who are likely to benefit most from chemoprophylaxis.

Impact of malaria chemoprophylaxis on the health of children in endemic areas

Only a few studies have investigated the impact of chemoprophylaxis on the health of young children in malaria-endemic areas and most have been small, controlled trials in which chemoprophylaxis was given under close supervision. The results of some of these studies are summarized in Table 1. In general, chemoprophylaxis led to a reduced incidence of clinical attacks of malaria, an

Table 1 The effects of malaria chemoprophylaxis on the health of children shown by small controlled trials undertaken in endemic areas of Africa. Significant results are shown in boldface

Year	Country	Age group (years)	Drug	Impact on health			Reference
				Clinical attacks	Nutrition	Hb/PCV	
1951–54	The Gambia	0–2	Chloroquine	—	↑Wt/age	↑**Hb**	McGregor et al. (1956)
1952	Gold Coast (Ghana)	12–20	Chloroquine	↓**School absences**	—	—	Wilson (cited in Colbourne, 1955)
1953–54	Gold Coast (Ghana)	7	Pyrimethamine	↓**School absences**	—	—	Colbourne (1955)
1953–54	Nigeria	5–10	Pyrimethamine	No change	↑**Wt**	No change	Archibald and Bruce-Chwatt (1956)
1966–67	Nigeria	8–17	Pyrimethamine + dapsone + sulphor-methoxine	↓**Clinic attendance**	—	↓**Anaemia**	Lucas et al. (1969)
1976–77	Mali	0–9	Chloroquine	—	—	No fall in PCV in rainy season	Delmont and Ranque (1981)
1976–79	Nigeria	0–2	Chloroquine	↓**68 % Clinical attacks**	↑Wt/age ↑Ht/age	↑**Hb** ↑**PCV**	Bradley-Moore et al. (1985a, 1985b, 1985c)
1976–79	Liberia	2–9	Chloroquine or chlorproguanil or pyrimethamine	↓**Fever episodes**	—	↑**PCV**	Björkman et al. (1986)

increase in haemoglobin (Hb) concentration or packed cell volume (PCV) and, in some trials, to a small increase in weight for age and/or height for age.

In 1972–1973 a large trial of chemoprophylaxis with pyrimethamine plus sulphalene was undertaken in northern Nigeria in 40 000 people (Molineaux and Gramiccia, 1980). Chemoprophylaxis was combined with regular indoor spraying with the residual insecticide propoxur. Highly effective malaria control was achieved by this combined approach and led to marked declines in infant and child mortality rates, both of which were very high before interventions were introduced. A reduction in the prevalence of fever was found and anthropometric measurements showed a small improvement in nutritional status among protected children.

During the 1980s a more modest control programme has been undertaken in The Gambia in which chemoprophylaxis has been given to about 1000 Gambian children under the age of 5 years over a period of several years. Maloprim (pyrimethamine + dapsone) was chosen for this trial because of concern that the use of chloroquine for chemoprophylaxis might encourage the emergence of parasites resistant to this drug, the mainstay of malaria treatment in The Gambia. Maloprim was given fortnightly throughout the rainy season by village health workers. The results of this study are summarized in Figure 1. Among children aged 1–4 years, but not in infants, there were marked reductions in the incidence of deaths overall, in the incidence of deaths attributed to malaria and in the incidence of clinical attacks of malaria detected by active surveillance (Greenwood *et al.*, 1988). PCVs were improved among the children who took prophylaxis. The protective effect of chemoprophylaxis was

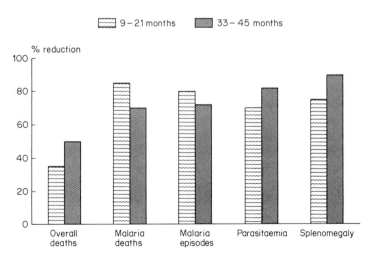

Figure 1   The levels of protection achieved from chemoprophylaxis in Gambian children aged 3–59 months, 9–21 months and 33–45 months after the start of a malaria chemoprophylaxis programme (from Menon *et al.*, 1990b)

sustained over a period of five years until the trial was stopped when it was considered to be unethical to continue (Menon *et al.*, 1990b).

The impact of malaria chemoprophylaxis on the outcome of pregnancy among women resident in malaria-endemic areas

Although it is recommended widely that women resident in malaria-endemic areas should take chemoprophylaxis during pregnancy there are few data to support this recommendation (Table 2). Malaria chemoprophylaxis with pyrimethamine or with the pyrimethamine combination Maloprim can increase the birth weight of infants born to primigravidae (Morley *et al.*, 1964; Greenwood *et al.*, 1989) but chloroquine proved to be less effective when used for this purpose in Nigeria (Gilles *et al.*, 1969) and Uganda (Hamilton *et al.*, 1972), despite the fact that the parasites prevalent in these areas at that time are likely to have been highly sensitive to chloroquine. In a more recent, large study undertaken in Malawi, chloroquine again had no significant effect on birth weight although a modest effect was obtained with mefloquine (Stekhetee *et al.*, unpublished). Although the results of this latest study may be accounted for by the increased prevalence of chloroquine-resistant parasites in East Africa they raise the possibility that chloroquine itself could have some effect on birth weight that counters its protective effect against malaria. It has never been demonstrated directly that chemoprophylaxis during pregnancy improves child survival but this is likely to be the case because birth weight is such a strong predictor of child survival. Data collected in The Gambia (Greenwood *et al.*, 1989) suggest that chemoprophylaxis might reduce mortality by about 50% among the infants of primigravidae.

Malaria can cause severe anaemia during pregnancy, especially in primigravidae, and studies in Nigeria (Fleming *et al.*, 1986), Kenya (Spencer *et al.*, 1987) and The Gambia (Greenwood *et al.*, 1989) have shown that chemoprophylaxis during pregnancy can reduce the incidence of anaemia in primigravidae.

The limited data available suggest that chemoprophylaxis has little influence on the outcome of pregnancy in multigravidae except among grand multigravidae (five pregnancies or more), among whom a significant increase in birth weight has been observed (Morley *et al.*, 1964; Greenwood *et al.*, 1989). Thus, it may be appropriate to target chemoprophylaxis at these two groups of pregnant women. Despite the seasonality of malaria in The Gambia the beneficial effects of chemoprophylaxis on birth weight were observed during both the dry season and the rainy season, in contrast to the effects of chemoprophylaxis on child survival.

Malaria chemoprophylaxis and migrants

It is likely that malaria chemoprophylaxis is used widely by employers in highly endemic areas to protect their workers on agricultural estates and on industrial

Table 2 The impact of malaria chemoprophylaxis on the outcome of pregnancy among women living in malaria-endemic areas. Significant results are shown in boldface

Year	Country	Drug	Effect on pregnancy		Reference
			Birth weight	Hb/PCV	
1963	Nigeria	Pyrimethamine	↑ **191 g para 0** ↑ **247 g para 4 +**	—	Morley et al. (1964)
1964–68	Nigeria	Chloroquine	↑ 85 g para 0	—	Gilles et al. (1969)
1965	Uganda	Chloroquine	↑ 40 g para 0	No effect	Hamilton et al. (1972)
?	Nigeria	Proguanil	—	↓ **Severe anaemia**	Fleming et al. (1986)
1983–84	Kenya	Chloroquine	—	↑ **Hb**	Spencer et al. (1987)
1984–87	The Gambia	Maloprim	↑ **159 g para 0** ↑ **93 g para 5 +**	↑ **PCV 3.5 %** **para 0**	Greenwood et al. (1989)

sites, such as mines, for example the LAMCO iron ore mine in Liberia (Bjorkman *et al.*, 1985a). However, little has been written about this aspect of chemoprophylaxis. Chemoprophylaxis may be especially important when workers move from an area of low to one of high endemicity, as may occur in Thailand (Kamolratanakul *et al.*, 1989) and in Brazil, where malaria has been a severe problem among migrants into parts of Amazonia.

The potential drawbacks to the use of malaria chemoprophylaxis in endemic areas

There are some potential drawbacks to the use of malaria chemoprophylaxis for the local populations of malaria-endemic areas which have led international organizations to discourage this form of malaria control (Table 3). However, although many of these objections are theoretically sound, few are based on solid experimental grounds. The following criticisms of chemoprophylaxis have been made.

Effective coverage of at-risk groups with chemoprophylaxis is difficult to achieve and impossible to sustain

In most endemic areas the at-risk groups who might be considered as candidates for chemoprophylaxis are young children and pregnant women. In the past delivery of chemoprophylaxis to a high proportion of young children and to pregnant women living in rural areas would have been difficult or impossible. However, many developing countries have now established primary health care (PHC) programmes based on village health workers (VHWs) and traditional birth attendants (TBAs) who can provide the means by which malaria chemoprophylaxis can be delivered to these at-risk groups (Haegman *et al.*, 1985; Greenwood *et al.*, 1988, 1989).

It is usually much easier to start than to sustain a new health intervention, and malaria chemoprophylaxis programmes are no exception to this rule; several programmes have expired after a promising start. MacCormack and Lwihula (1983) investigated the reasons behind the failure of a large malaria chemopro-phylaxis study involving 100 000 children in North Mara, Tanzania. Various

Table 3 Potential drawbacks to chemoprophylaxis as a malaria control strategy

(1)	Chemoprophylaxis is difficult to sustain
(2)	Chemoprophylaxis is expensive
(3)	Chemoprophylaxis is dangerous
(4)	Chemoprophylaxis impairs the development of natural immunity to malaria
(5)	Chemoprophylaxis encourages the spread of drug-resistant parasites

problems were identified, including failures of drug supply, lack of understanding of the purpose of the trial and a high incidence of vomiting and itching
induced by chloroquine which was used as the chemoprophylactic agent.
Ensuring a regular supply of prophylactic drug is likely to be a major difficulty
in many areas but may be possible when there is an effective system for
delivering curative drugs to PHC workers.

Experience in The Gambia shows that progressive lack of compliance with
chemoprophylaxis is not inevitable. Thus, in about one-third of the villages in
the Farafenni study area, high levels of drug administration were maintained
over a period of five years despite little reinforcement (Allen *et al.*, 1990c)
(Figure 2). However, in another one-third of the villages levels of drug administration declined progressively. As expected, the programme was most effective in

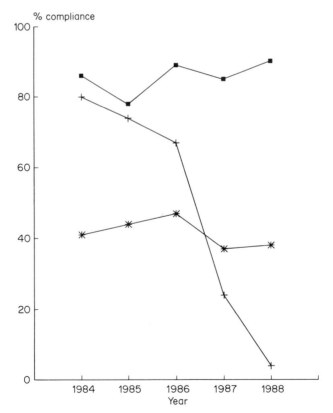

Figure 2 Compliance with malaria chemoprophylaxis in three representative Gambian
villages over a five-year period. Compliance is expressed as the number of occasions on
which a drug was given as a percentage of the number of occasions on which it should
have been administered by a village health worker (from Allen *et al.*, 1990c)

villages with a strong head, political unity and a well-motivated VHW. Appreciation by mothers of the benefits of chemoprophylaxis was another important factor that sustained the programme in these communities. Nevertheless, it is clear that in most communities chemoprophylaxis will not be sustained unless there is a continuing process of education and encouragement.

Chemoprophylaxis is too expensive to sustain

The costs of a chemoprophylaxis programme will vary from community to community depending on the availability of a suitable drug delivery system, the nature of the drug that is to be used and the size of the at-risk groups. Costs need not necessarily be high. Thus, in The Gambia, where VHWs are supported by their village and where the health authorities have established a system for the delivery of curative drugs to VHWs, the major cost of chemoprophylaxis to the health services is that of the drug itself. The costs of giving Maloprim weekly to children for 20 weeks during the period of maximum malaria transmission in The Gambia are in the region of US$0.6 per child per year or US$3 per child for the first five years of life, a figure that compares favourably with the approximate amount of US$15 required for full immunization. A rough estimate suggests that, in The Gambia, the cost of each life saved by malaria chemoprophylaxis is in the region of US$30.

Although drug costs in this range are modest it is unlikely that they could be met for a prolonged period by the health services of a poor developing country and likely that drug costs for such a programme would have to be covered either by aid or by some form of cost-recovery system.

Chemoprophylaxis is dangerous

All drugs used for malaria chemoprophylaxis have some side-effects and these may occasionally be serious and even fatal. The incidence of serious side-effects associated with the use of drugs such as Fansidar and Maloprim for chemoprophylaxis is about 1 in 20 000 for Caucasian visitors to endemic areas but it is not known whether this figure applies also to the resident populations of these countries. Nevertheless, it must be accepted that if drugs such as Maloprim are used for prophylaxis on a large scale they will cause serious reactions occasionally and, perhaps, even deaths. Whether this is acceptable will depend on the severity of the malaria situation that they are being used to prevent.

Many antimalarial drugs produce minor side-effects in a significant proportion of subjects. In African populations chloroquine frequently causes severe itching and this, together with its bitter taste, has been an important factor in discouraging the regular use of chloroquine as a chemoprophylactic in many African communities (MacCormack and Lwihula, 1983).

Chemoprophylaxis impairs the development of natural immunity to malaria

The possibility that long-term administration of chemoprophylaxis might impair the development of natural immunity to malaria has been one of the main reasons for resistance to this form of malaria control—there would be little point in saving a child from death from malaria during the first few years of life if he or she were to die from malaria shortly after chemoprophylaxis was stopped. There can be little doubt that when given extremely conscientiously malaria chemoprophylaxis will interfere with the development of malaria immunity, for example in expatriates resident in malaria-endemic areas. However, whether this is the case when malaria chemoprophylaxis is given under field conditions is much less certain.

Concerns about the possible impact of chemoprophylaxis on the development of protective immunity were enhanced by the results of several early studies which showed that children who received malaria chemoprophylaxis had lower titres of antimalarial antibodies than control children (Table 4). However, in these early studies, antibody levels were measured by immunofluorescent antibody tests (IFAT) or other simple assays which reflect only exposure and which provide little or no information about protective immunity. Therefore, in a recent study, Otoo *et al.* (1988 and unpublished) measured levels of a variety of antibodies, some with defined biological functions which may be related to protective immunity, in Gambian children who had received chemoprophylaxis with Maloprim for a variable number of years and in control children from the same communities (Figure 3). Some differences were found between children in the two groups but, in general, these were not marked. The results of this study and those of a previous trial undertaken in Nigeria (Bradley-Moore *et al.*, 1985a) have shown that differences between control and protected children diminish the longer that chemoprophylaxis is given (Figure 3).

During the recent study undertaken in The Gambia, cell-mediated immune responses to malaria antigens were measured as well as antibody titres. Proliferative and γ-interferon responses were higher in children who were receiving prophylaxis than in control children (Otoo *et al.*, 1989). The probable explanation for this apparently paradoxical finding is that because these children had been exposed to less frequent and less heavy malaria infections than the controls they had been able to overcome some of the suppressive effects of malaria on cell-mediated immunity and thus to develop a good immune response to malaria antigens.

Because there is no clearly defined immunological marker for protective immunity to malaria, studies of the kind described above can give only limited information about the effects of chemoprophylaxis on protective immunity. Definitive results can come only from studies in which protective immunity is measured by direct observation; few attempts have been made to do this. In 1966 Pringle and Avery-Jones reported an increase in the severity of malaria infections in a group of Tanzanian schoolchildren after a single dose of

Table 4 The influence of malaria chemoprophylaxis on the immune response to malarial antigens

Year	Country	Age group (years)	Drug	Duration of chemo-prophylaxis (years)	Change in immune response Humoral	Change in immune response Cellular	Reference
1952–57	The Gambia	3–5	Chloroquine	3–5	↓γ-Globulin		McGregor and Gilles (1960)
1963	The Gambia	<1	Pyrimethamine	<1	↓IFAT antibody		Voller and Wilson (1964)
1971–74	Uganda	2–3	Pyrimethamine	2–3	↓IFAT antibody		Harland et al. (1975)
1972–73	Nigeria	All	Pyrimethamine + sulfalene	1	↓IFAT antibody ↓IHA antibody ↓Precipitin antibody		Cornille Brogger et al. (1978)
1976–79	Nigeria	1–2	Chloroquine	1–2	↓IFAT antibody ↓ELISA antibody		Bradley-Moore et al. (1985a)
1981–82	Burkina Faso	0–10	Chloroquine	1–2	↓IFAT antibody		Brandicourt et al. (1987)
1983–88	The Gambia	0–5	Maloprim	0–5	↓Many antibodies	↑Proliferation γ-interferon production	Otoo et al., (1988, 1989)

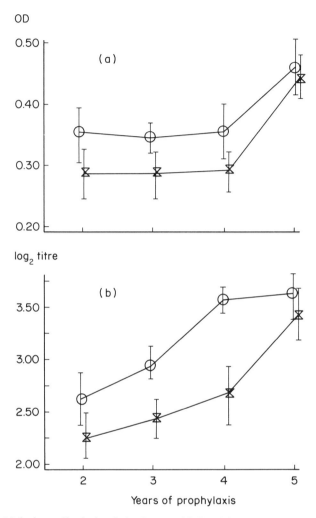

Figure 3   Malaria antibody levels in 5-year-old Gambian children who had received malaria chemoprophylaxis ⊠ or placebo ◯ for two to five years previously. (a) ELISA antibodies against an antigen prepared from a *P. falciparum*-infected placenta. (b) IFAT antibodies to *P. falciparum*. (Otoo *et al.*, unpublished results)

chloroquine and three, weekly treatments with primaquine. This observation is quoted widely as evidence for loss of protective immunity following prophylaxis. However, the conclusions of this study are based on the finding that parasite densities were higher in blood films collected from study schoolchildren during a four-week period after treatment than in pre-treatment blood films. No contemporary controls were studied, so that the significance of this finding is very uncertain. In another study undertaken in schoolchildren, Archibald and Bruce-Chwatt (1956) did not find any significant increase in absences from school during a three-month period after study children had received chemoprophylaxis with pyrimethamine for two years. In a community study undertaken in young children in Nigeria Bradley-Moore *et al.* (1985a) observed no rebound in mortality or morbidity after two years of chemoprophylaxis with chloroquine and, in Liberia, Bjorkman *et al.* (1986) found no rebound in fever attacks after two years of chemoprophylaxis with pyrimethamine or chlorproguanil; equi vocal results were obtained after chemoprophylaxis with chloroquine. Similarly, in the large Garki study, no clear indication for a rebound in mortality or morbidity was found after the intervention was stopped (Molineaux and Gramiccia, 1980).

The possibility that stopping chemoprophylaxis might be followed by a rebound in mortality and morbidity has been investigated carefully in the recent study undertaken in The Gambia. Children were visited weekly for one year after chemoprophylaxis was stopped and mortality surveillance has been maintained subsequently. No rebound in the incidence of clinical attacks of malaria was seen between the ages of 5 and 6 years in children who had received prophylaxis for one to four years previously. However, there was a significant increase in the incidence of clinical attacks of malaria among children who had received prophylaxis from the age of 3 months to 5 years (Figure 4) (Otoo *et al.*,

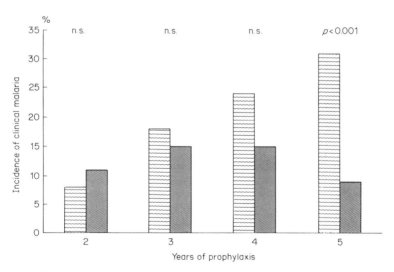

Figure 4 The incidence of clinical attacks of malaria (fever + malaria parasitaemia) in Gambian children during a one-year period after they had stopped taking chemoprophylaxis or placebo at the age of 5 years according to the duration for which drug administration had been received. ▨, children who had received chemoprophylaxis; ▨, children who had received placebo (Otoo *et al.*, unpublished results)

unpublished). No evidence for a rebound in mortality on stopping chemoprophylaxis was found; the mortality rate among children aged 6–10 years who had
received prophylaxis for varying periods up to the age of 5 years was similar to
that found in children who had not (Alonso *et al.*, unpublished). However, the
number of deaths among children in this age group was small and consequently
the power of the study to detect a rebound effect on mortality was low.

Overall, there is little to suggest that when given in field conditions chemoprophylaxis impairs substantially the development of protective immunity. The
probable reason for this is that prophylaxis is not completely effective and that
children who are supposed to be protected experience occasional breakthrough
infections. Thus, the prevalence of parasitaemia in children receiving chloroquine prophylaxis under close supervision in Nigeria was 9% (Bradley-Moore
et al., 1985a) and that in those receiving Maloprim in The Gambia 11%
(Greenwood *et al.*, 1988). Occasional infections such as these may be as effective
at inducing protective immunity as repeated and heavy exposure.

Chemoprophylaxis and the spread of drug resistance

Another major concern with regard to the widespread use of chemoprophylaxis
in endemic areas is that it may encourage the emergence and spread of drug-
resistant parasites. This is a reasonable supposition but it is one for which there
is only limited evidence. It has been reported on several occasions that when
pyrimethamine has been used alone for prophylaxis pyrimethamine-resistant
isolates have emerged rapidly (Clyde and Shute, 1957; Michel, 1961). However,
in the case of chloroquine the position is much less clear. The use of chloro-
quine-impregnated salt and of chloroquine tablets for prophylaxis over a period
of many years has been blamed for the emergence and spread of chloroquine-
resistant *P. falciparum* in northern Tanzania (Onori *et al.*, 1982; Draper *et al.*,
1985) but chloroquine-resistant parasites appeared at about the same time in
other areas of East Africa where chemoprophylaxis had not been used.
Furthermore, chloroquine resistance has been slow to emerge in the large cities
of West Africa where antimalarials have been available freely for many years
and are consumed widely. In The Gambia chloroquine resistance appeared first
in the centre of the country, not in the areas near to the capital where
chloroquine is used most frequently (Menon *et al.*, 1990a). Nevertheless, it must
be accepted as probable that widespread use of an antimalarial for chemoprophylaxis will encourage the spread of parasites resistant to the drug once
these have emerged.

A possible way of postponing this serious complication of chemoprophylaxis
is to restrict prophylaxis to only those groups most at risk, thus reducing drug
pressure on the parasite. There is some evidence that this approach can work.
Thus, in Liberia, Bjorkman *et al.* (1985b) found no resistance to chlorproguanil
even after the drug had been used for chemoprophylaxis in village children for

seven years. Similarly, in The Gambia, targeted chemoprophylaxis with chlor-proguanil or Maloprim for five years did not lead to an increase in the prevalence of parasites resistant to these drugs (Allen *et al.*, 1990a, 1990b).

The possible role for malaria chemoprophylaxis in the protection of the resident populations of malaria-endemic areas in the 1990s

There is now good evidence that malaria chemoprophylaxis can be given effectively to at-risk groups by PHC workers and that it can have a major impact on the health of young children and primigravidae. It is also clear that some of the disadvantages of chemoprophylaxis are not as serious as had once been feared. Thus, in some circumstances, chemoprophylaxis may be an appropriate method of malaria control for high-risk groups resident in malaria-endemic areas. However, before a decision is made to use chemoprophylaxis in any target group a stringent assessment of its potential benefits and risks must be made. This can be done only when the pattern of malaria in the community in question has been defined carefully. Some of the variables that must be taken into consideration are shown in Figure 5.

In situations where a small proportion of the population is at high risk from severe or fatal malaria and where relatively safe drugs are still effective, a strong case for targeted chemoprophylaxis can be made. The Gambia and similar communities where as many as one in 20 children still die from malaria may be such a case. In contrast, parts of South-East Asia where a high proportion of the population are at relatively low risk of infection and where the prevalent parasite is highly resistant to antimalarials are not candidates for a malaria chemoprophylaxis programme. In many epidemiological situations it is more difficult to balance benefits and risks. However, the spread of drug-resistant *P. falciparum* is swinging the balance against the use of malaria chemoprophylaxis as an appropriate malaria control measure for even high-risk groups in many malaria endemic areas.

In the future chemoprophylaxis may be found to have a useful role to play in the protection of high-risk groups when used in combination with another partially effective malaria control measure such as insecticide-impregnated bednets or a malaria vaccine which gives only partial protection. Insecticide-impregnated bednets, considered on pp. 67–82, are an exciting new development but they are only partially effective at preventing clinical attacks of malaria, even when used under optimal circumstances (Rozendaal, 1989). Thus, we have investigated recently the effects of using chemoprophylaxis in combination with insecticide-impregnated bednets. Addition of chemoprophylaxis, given during the peak malaria transmission season, did not give young children any addition-al protection against death over that provided by impregnated nets alone, but clinical attacks of malaria were reduced by 95% in children who received

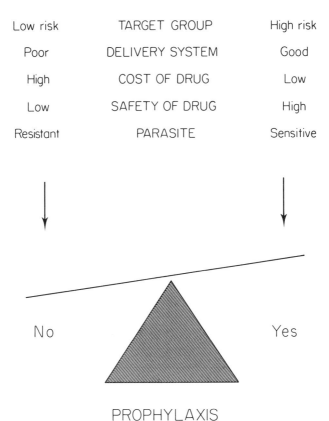

Low risk	TARGET GROUP	High risk
Poor	DELIVERY SYSTEM	Good
High	COST OF DRUG	Low
Low	SAFETY OF DRUG	High
Resistant	PARASITE	Sensitive

No   Yes

PROPHYLAXIS

Figure 5   Factors to be considered in deciding whether to use malaria chemoprophylaxis

Table 5   The influence of insecticide-impregnated bednets alone and
combined with chemoprophylaxis with Maloprim on the incidence of
clinical malaria and on the prevalence of malaria infection in Gambian
children aged 6–59 months

Intervention	Clinical attacks per 1000 weeks at risk	Parasitaemia (%)
Nets plus chemoprophylaxis	1.3	3
Nets alone	12.0	26
Controls	24.6	43

Alonso *et al.* (unpublished).

chemoprophylaxis and slept under impregnated nets but only 51 % in those who slept under impregnated bednets alone (Alonso *et al.*, unpublished) (Table 5). Chemoprophylaxis can prevent mortality and morbidity from malaria among the resident population of malaria-endemic areas but it should be used only in circumstances in which careful assessment indicates that its benefits are likely to outweigh its potential harmful effects.

Acknowledgements

The support of the many scientists who have contributed to the Farafenni project and the encouragement of the Medical and Health Department of the Government of The Gambia for this project are acknowledged gratefully.

References

Allen SJ, Otoo LN, Cooke GA, O'Donnell A and Greenwood BM (1990a) Sensitivity of *Plasmodium falciparum* to chlorproguanil in Gambian children after five years of continuous prophylaxis. *Transactions of the Royal Society of Tropical Medicine and Hygiene, 84,* 218

Allen SJ, Otoo LN, Cooke JA, O'Donnell A and Greenwood BM (1990b) Sensitivity of *Plasmodium falciparum* to Maloprim after five years of targeted chemoprophylaxis in a rural area of The Gambia. *Transactions of the Royal Society of Tropical Medicine and Hygiene, 84,* 666–667

Allen SJ, Snow RW, Menon A and Greenwood BM (1990c) Compliance with malaria chemoprophylaxis over a five-year period among children in a rural area of The Gambia. *Journal of Tropical Medicine and Hygiene, 93,* 313–322

Archibald HM and Bruce-Chwatt LJ (1956) Suppression of malaria with pyrimethamine in Nigerian schoolchildren. *Bulletin of the World Health Organization, 15,* 775–784

Björkman A, Hedman P, Broholt J, Willcox M, Diamant I, Pehrson PO, Rombo L and Bengtsson E (1985a) Different malaria control activities in an area of Liberia: effects on malariometric parameters. *Annals of Tropical Medicine and Parasitology, 79,* 239–246

Björkman A, Broholt J, Willcox M, Pehrson PO, Rombo L, Hedman P, Hetland G, Kollie E, Hanson AP and Bengtsson E (1985b) Malaria control by chlorproguanil. 1. Clinical effects and susceptibility of *Plasmodium falciparum in vivo* after seven years of monthly chlorproguanil administration to children in a Liberian village. *Annals of Tropical Medicine and Parasitology, 79,* 597–601

Björkman A, Broholt J, Pehrson PO, Willcox M, Rombo L, Hedman P, Kollie E, Alestig K, Hanson A and Bengtsson E (1986) Monthly antimalarial chemotherapy to children in a holoendemic area of Liberia. *Annals of Tropical Medicine and Parasitology, 80,* 155–167

Bradley-Moore AM, Greenwood BM, Bradley AK, Bartlett A, Bidwell DE, Voller A, Kirkwood BR and Gilles HM (1985a) Malaria chemoprophylaxis with chloroquine in young Nigerian children. I. Its effects on mortality, morbidity and the prevalence of malaria. *Annals of Tropical Medicine and Parasitology, 79,* 549–562

Bradley-Moore AM, Greenwood BM, Bradley AK, Kirkwood BR and Gilles HM (1985b) Malaria chemoprophylaxis with chloroquine in young Nigerian children. III. Its effect on nutrition. *Annals of Tropical Medicine and Parasitology, 79,* 575–584

Bradley-Moore AM, Greenwood BM, Bradley AK, Akintunde A, Attai EDE, Fleming

AF, Flynn FV, Kirkwood BR and Gilles HM (1985c) Malaria chemoprophylaxis with chloroquine in young Nigerian children. IV. Its effect on haematological measurements. *Annals of Tropical Medicine and Parasitology, 79,* 585–595

Brandicourt O, Carnevale P, Baudon D, Molez JF, Gazin P, Danis M, Duflo B and Gentilini M (1987) Influence de la chimioprophylaxie ou de la chimiotherapie par la chloroquine sur l'acquisition des anticorps fluorescents antipalustres en zonede savane. *Bulletin de la Société Belgique de Médecine Tropicale, 67,* 17–22

Cavalie P and Mouchet J (1962) Les campagnes experimentales d'eradication du paludisme dans le nord de la république du Cameroun. *Médecine Tropicale, 22,* 95–118

Clyde DF and Shute GT (1957) Resistance of *Plasmodium falciparum* in Tanganyika to pyrimethamine administered at weekly intervals. *Transactions of the Royal Society of Tropical Medicine and Hygiene, 51,* 505–513

Colbourne MJ (1955) The effect of malaria suppression in a group of Accra school children. *Transactions of the Royal Society of Tropical Medicine and Hygiene, 49,* 356–369

Cornille Brogger R, Mathews HM, Storey J, Ashkar TS, Brogger S and Molineaux L (1978) Changing patterns in the humoral immune response to malaria before, during, and after the application of control measures: a longitudinal study in the West African savanna. *Bulletin of the World Health Organization, 56,* 579–600

Delmont J and Ranque P (1981) Influence d'une chimioprophylaxie antipaludique sur l'etat de santé d'une communaute rurale en Afrique de L'Ouest. *Bulletin de la Société de Pathologie Exotique, 74,* 600–610

Draper CC, Brubaker G, Geser A, Kilimali VAEB and Wernsdorfer WH (1985) Serial studies on the evolution of chloroquine resistance in an area of East Africa receiving intermittent malaria chemosuppression. *Bulletin of the World Health Organization, 63,* 109–118

Escudie A, Hamon J and Schneider J (1962) Resultats d'une chimoprophylaxie antipaludique de masse par l'association amino-4-quinoleine/amino-8-quinoleine en milieu rural African de la region de Bobo-Dioulasso (Haute-Volta) 1960. *Médecine Tropicale, 22,* 268–305

Fleming AF, Ghatoura GBS, Harrison KA, Briggs ND and Dunn DT (1986) The prevention of anaemia in pregnancy in primigravidae in the guinea savanna of Nigeria. *Annals of Tropical Medicine and Parasitology, 80,* 211–233

Garfield RM and Vermund SH (1983) Changes in malaria incidence after mass drug administration in Nicaragua. *Lancet, ii,* 500–503

Gilles HM, Lawson JB, Sibelas M, Voller A and Allan N (1969) Malaria, anaemia and pregnancy. *Annals of Tropical Medicine and Parasitology, 63,* 245–263

Greenwood BM, Greenwood AM, Bradley AK, Snow RW, Byass P, Hayes RJ and N'Jie ABH (1988) Comparison of two strategies for control of malaria within a primary health care programme in The Gambia. *Lancet, i,* 1121–1127

Greenwood BM, Greenwood AM, Snow RW, Byass P, Bennett S and Hatib-N'Jie AB (1989) The effects of malaria chemoprophylaxis given by traditional birth attendants on the course and outcome of pregnancy. *Transactions of the Royal Society of Tropical Medicine and Hygiene, 83,* 589–594

Haegman F, Wyffels A and Alzouma G (1985) Malaria control by village health workers in the province of Dosso, Niger. Part 1. Operational analysis. *Annales de la Société Belge de Médecine Tropicale, 65,* 17–144

Hamilton PJS, Gebbie DAM, Wilks NE and Lothe F (1972) The role of malaria, folic acid deficiency and haemoglobin AS in pregnancy at Mulago Hospital. *Transactions of the Royal Society of Tropical Medicine and Hygiene, 66,* 594–602

Harland PSEG, Frood JD and Parkin JM (1975) Some effects of partial malaria suppression in Ugandan children during the first 3 years of life. *Transactions of the Royal Society of Tropical Medicine and Hygiene*, 69, 261–262

Kamolratanakul P, Viputsiri O, Dhanamun B, Hirunabut S, Mekmasin A and Thongsawat P (1989) The effectiveness of chemoprophylaxis against malaria for non-immune migrant workers in eastern Thailand. *Transactions of the Royal Society of Tropical Medicine and Hygiene*, 83, 313–315

Lucas AO, Hendrickse RG, Okubadejo OA, Richards WHG, Neal RA and Kofie BAK (1969) The suppression of malarial parasitaemia by pyrimethamine in combination with dapsone or sulphormethoxine. *Transactions of the Royal Society of Tropical Medicine and Hygiene*, 63, 216–229

MacCormack CP and Lwihula G (1983) Failure to participate in a malaria chemosuppression programme: North Mara, Tanzania. *Journal of Tropical Medicine and Hygiene*, 86, 99–107

McGregor IA and Gilles HM (1960) Studies on the significance of high serum gamma-globulin concentrations in Gambian Africans. II. Gamma-globulin concentrations of Gambian children in the fourth, fifth and sixth years of life. *Annals of Tropical Medicine and Parasitology*, 54, 275–280

McGregor IA, Gilles HM, Walters JH, Davies AH and Pearson FA (1956) Effects of heavy and repeated malaria infections on Gambian infants and children. *British Medical Journal, ii*, 686–692

Menon A, Otoo LN, Herbage EA and Greenwood BM (1990a) A national survey of the prevalence of chloroquine resistant *Plasmodium falciparum* malaria in The Gambia. *Transactions of the Royal Society of Tropical Medicine and Hygiene*, 84, 638–640

Menon A, Snow RW, Byass P, Greenwood BM, Hayes RJ and N'Jie ABH (1990b) Sustained protection against mortality and morbidity from malaria in rural Gambian children by chemoprophylaxis given by village health workers. *Transactions of the Royal Society of Tropical Medicine and Hygiene*, 84, 768–772

Michel R (1961) Resistance à la pyrimethamine dans la zone antipaludique de Thiès (Senegal). *Médecine Tropicale*, 21, 876–878

Molineaux L and Gramiccia G (1980) *The Garki Project*. World Health Organization, Geneva

Morley D, Woodland M and Cuthbertson WFJ (1964) Controlled trial of pyrimethamine in pregnant women in an African village. *British Medical Journal, i*, 667–668

Onori E, Payne D, Grab B, Horst HI, Almeida Franco J and Joia H (1982) Incipient resistance of *Plasmodium falciparum* to chloroquine among a semi-immune population of the United Republic of Tanzania. 1. Results of *in vivo* and *in vitro* studies and of an ophthalmological survey. *Bulletin of the World Health Organization*, 60, 77–87

Otoo LN, Snow RW, Menon A, Byass P and Greenwood BM (1988) Immunity to malaria in young Gambian children after a two-year period of chemoprophylaxis. *Transactions of the Royal Society of Tropical Medicine and Hygiene*, 82, 59–65

Otoo LN, Riley EM, Menon A, Byass P and Greenwood BM (1989) Cellular immune responses to *Plasmodium falciparum* antigens in children receiving long-term anti-malarial chemoprophylaxis. *Transactions of the Royal Society of Tropical Medicine and Hygiene*, 83, 778–782

Pringle G and Avery-Jones S (1966) Observations on the early course of untreated falciparum malaria in semi-immune African children following a short period of protection. *Bulletin of the World Health Organization*, 34, 269–272

Ransford O (1983) '*Bid the Sickness Cease*'. Murray, London

Rozendaal JA (1989) Impregnated mosquito nets and curtains for self protection and vector control. *Tropical Diseases Bulletin*, *86*, R1–R41

Spencer HC, Kaseje DCO, Sempebwa EKN, Huong AY and Roberts JM (1987) Malaria chemoprophylaxis to pregnant women provided by community health workers in Saradidi, Kenya. II. Effect on parasitaemia and haemoglobin levels. *Annals of Tropical Medicine and Parasitology*, *81*, (Suppl. 1), 83–89

Voller A and Wilson H (1964) Immunological aspects of a population under prophylaxis against malaria. *British Medical Journal*, *ii*, 551–552

WORKSHOP REPORT AND RECOMMENDATIONS
RAPPORTEUR: BERNARD J. BRABIN

Several general considerations should guide decisions about the use of anti-malarial chemoprophylaxis in populations living in endemic areas. The first is that chemoprophylaxis is not an alternative to treatment. It is, however, important to consider whether prophylaxis would be beneficial in addition to treatment. It follows that prophylaxis should not be considered unless some infrastructure is in place to provide treatment.

Malaria-specific mortality rates in children are needed for estimates of the magnitude of the problem. The incidence rates of severe malaria and cerebral malaria would also be useful indicators. In areas where these are high the adequacy of treatment facilities must be ensured and the potential benefits of prophylaxis assessed for target groups. For pregnant women the population-attributable risk of low birth weight in primiparae due to malaria could prove a useful indicator (Brabin, 1991).

The degree of misuse or overuse of drugs is a major concern. Mass drug usage should be avoided except in special circumstances such as focal epidemics. Only high-risk groups should be targeted and essentially these are pregnant women and young children. Caution against the overuse of drugs will be required if inadequate evidence is available of their benefits. The sustainability of a chemoprophylaxis programme must be addressed from the outset and malaria-specific mortality rates could be used' to guide success. Information and operational research are required about current chemoprophylaxis programmes with regard to how well they have been sustained and the rebound effects if the programmes are discontinued. Monitoring for drug resistance should be included as part of the programme.

What are the specific situations in which prophylaxis is desirable? In populations where intense transmission occurs, which may include certain forest-fringe dwellers, high-risk groups only should be targeted (young children and pregnant women). If malaria is markedly seasonal, use should be limited to the peak transmission period. Populations such as military personnel, migrant groups and refugees need special consideration. In refugee camps prophylaxis should be time-limited but is necessary even if treatment facilities are poor, as time may be required to develop the necessary infrastructure. Irrigation scheme workers could be at special risk and, for these, treatment facilities should be available although short-term prophylaxis could be advantageous for seasonal settlements. In urban areas treatment facilities should be the mainstay for management.

Drug choice is limited because specific drugs need to be reserved for treatment. However, the stage has been passed for chloroquine to be withheld from use for chemoprophylaxis on the grounds that it should be kept in reserve for treatment. Chloroquine, proguanil and Maloprim are the primary drugs for prophylaxis, but quinine, artemesinine, halofantrine, mefloquine and Fansidar should be reserved for treatment. Mefloquine could be considered as a prophylactic in pregnancy, except in the first trimester, in areas with a high degree of chloroquine resistance.

The infrastructure needed and supervision which must be established and maintained to ensure a workable delivery system to PHC workers offering drugs are stressed. These aspects include attention to the logistics of drug supply and development of an essential drug list. The cost of sustaining such programmes depends on external funding as it is unlikely these could be wholly paid by government. The economics of maintainance of treatment and chemoprophylaxis should be an area specified for donor support. The role of the community in understanding, supporting and maintaining a programme and in generating income to cover costs is crucial. With the widespread use of drugs information is required on their adverse effects so as to encourage clearer recommendations from manufacturers. This information is more easily obtained in urban areas.

Integral to the success of chemoprophylaxis would be a monitoring and evaluation system. As long as the mortality risks remain high, despite the provision of treatment facilities, then a prophylaxis programme would need to be sustained. When that programme is discontinued special attention will be required to ensure adequate treatment is available; there should be a strong educational component about treatment when chemoprophylaxis is stopped as the risks of rebound morbidity may be unforeseen.

The issue of chemoprophylaxis in pregnancy raises several questions. Prophylaxis should probably be recommended for all pregnant women as evidence from recent field studies has demonstrated significant benefits especially in terms of reduction in the prevalence of low birth weight and maternal anaemia. However, concern has been raised over the feasibility of implementing this recommendation as compliance issues are unresolved and chloroquine resistance may significantly reduce potential benefits. But, the benefits related to reducing maternal anaemia should not be underestimated as this has been achieved even in areas with substantial chloroquine resistance at RI level and maternal anaemia has been associated with increased low birth-weight risk in primiparae (Brabin *et al.*, 1990). Operational research assessing daily compliance with prophylactic use of proguanil would assist in resolving the issue of daily prophylaxis in pregnancy. Anecdotal evidence for compliance with daily proguanil is reported and in a recent field trial in Tanzania improved efficacy was achieved in pregnant women when daily proguanil was given (W. Kilama, personal communication). Mefloquine is available as a second-line prophylactic in pregnant women. Research issues that remain to be resolved include an assessment of malaria risk in second pregnancies of women taking chemoprophylaxis as primigravidae.

There are indications that rebound clinical malaria occurs with increasing frequency in relation to duration of chemoprophylaxis. Shorter periods of prophylaxis are therefore preferable and the duration could be governed by age-specific malaria mortality in young children. On clinical grounds 5 years is suggested to be a useful age to discontinue as by then most children could communicate readily if they develop malaria symptoms. Information is required on the effects of malaria chemoprophylaxis in infants and the consequences on morbidity and mortality if discontinued prematurely. Its effects on the gametocyte rate are unknown.

References

Brabin BJ (1991) An assessment of low birthweight risk in primiparae as an indicator of malaria control in pregnancy. *International Journal of Epidemiology*, *20*, 276–283
Brabin BJ, Brabin L, Sapau J and Galme K (1990) Consequences of maternal anaemia on outcome of pregnancy in a malaria endemic area in Papua New Guinea. *Annals of Tropical Medicine and Parasitology*, *84*, 11–24

Drug resistance—changing patterns

Anders Björkman

Karolinska Institute, Stockholm, Sweden

Introduction

Resistance of *Plasmodium falciparum* (Pf) to chloroquine and other existing antimalarial drugs represents a major obstacle to malaria control today. This chapter summarizes the present epidemiological situation of drug resistance and its changing patterns, considers its determinants and implications, including lessons learnt from past activities, and makes recommendations for future policies.

Epidemiology of drug resistance

Dihydrofolate reductase inhibitors ('antifols')

Antifols have been mainly considered as causal prophylactic drugs, although pyrimethamine has been used also in combination with sulfadoxine for therapy. Resistance to pyrimethamine soon develops and for many years has been widespread in most endemic areas (Peters, 1987). Pyrimethamine alone is therefore not advocated for prophylatic use. The protective efficacy of proguanil is difficult to estimate owing to lack of controlled studies. In Thailand an efficacy of about 50% has been obtained (Pang *et al.*, 1989; Limsomwong *et al.*, 1988). In Africa its efficacy has mainly been studied in surveys of travellers and an efficacy of the same order as that in Thailand has been shown recently (Phillips-Howard *et al.*, 1990). It has long been assumed that proguanil and chlorproguanil would quickly induce resistance in the same way as pyrimethamine. However, studies in Liberia (Björkman, 1985a) and in The Gambia (Allen *et al.*, 1990) show little if any resistance to chlorproguanil even after several years of regular use by a significant number of people. The reasons for the difference between chlorproguanil (proguanil) and pyrimethamine in this respect remain unclear. The effect of withdrawal of pyrimethamine from a resistant area has been studied in Tanzania with conflicting results. From follow-up studies in an area where pyrimethamine was used, sensitivity increased again in the absence of drug pressure (Clyde, 1967). However, in an adjacent area, pyrimethamine-resistant parasites were still abundant 15 years later (Kouznetsov *et al.*, 1980). When pyrimethamine was withdrawn from a drug-resistant focus in Liberia, there was an initial reduction of resistance during the first two years but the level remained similar for the next eight years (Björkman, 1985, and unpublished).

Cross-resistance between antifols has been shown *in vitro* for the blood stages of Pf, although not consistently, and recent genetic findings suggest different mutation sites for pyrimethamine and cycloguanil, the active metabolite of proguanil (Foote *et al.*, 1990; Peterson *et al.*, 1990). Also, whereas the activity of pyrimethamine was reduced 750-fold against resistant isolates, the corresponding reduction for cycloguanil was only 7.7-fold (Watkins *et al.*, 1987). Since its causal prophylactic efficacy is stronger than the therapeutic effect, proguanil may thus still provide protection against less sensitive strains.

One intriguing issue has been the large individual variation in the metabolism of proguanil into the active metabolite, cycloguanil (Ward *et al.*, 1989), which suggests that some individuals would be less protected from Pf infections by proguanil than others. However, eight non-immune Swedish subjects in Guinea-Bissau (Björkman *et al.*, unpublished results) and 13 semi-immune school-children in Kenya (Ward *et al.*, 1989) with Pf breakthrough during proguanil prophylaxis did not differ significantly in their proguanil/cycloguanil ratio from the control subjects who had not experienced Pf infections.

A similar compound to proguanil, chlorproguanil, has an active metabolite, chlorcycloguanil, which has proved to be more active than cycloguanil. Although the elimination half-life is not significantly different from that of proguanil, chlorproguanil has been recommended in a weekly dose, which probably is the main reason for failures in recent trials.

The relatively shorter elimination half-life and higher efficacy of proguanil (and chlorproguanil) than pyrimethamine has prompted its use in combination with potentiating sulpha drugs of similar short-elimination half-life and thus possibly with less risk of serious adverse reactions than drugs with long half-lives such as sulfadoxine (Björkman and Phillips-Howard, 1991). In two recent studies such a prophylactic combination showed five- to ten-fold reduction of Pf incidence compared with proguanil alone in South-East Asia (Pang *et al.*, 1989; Karwacki *et al.*, 1990). The combination of proguanil or chlorproguanil with sulpha drugs may also prove to be valuable in the treatment of Pf infection, and indeed a few recent trials have shown promising results (Watkins *et al.*, 1988; Keuter *et al.*, 1990).

Chloroquine

Chloroquine-resistant Pf (CRPf) has now spread to all but a few isolated areas with Pf malaria. During the 1960s and 1970s, resistance became established in most of South-East Asia and South America, and during the 1980s in most of Africa. The evolution of CRPf is more fulminant in South-East Asia than in South America and the frequencies of resistant parasites in different areas still

vary, especially in Africa. Here recent *in vitro* studies showed that between 10%
and 90% of Pf isolates were drug resistant and similar findings of drug failures *in
vivo* were made (Björkman and Phillips-Howard, 1990), although in many areas
partial protective immunity may assist in the *in vivo* clearance of resistant
parasites. The clinical efficacy may be adequate in those with a partial immunity
even if the parasites do only partly respond to the treatment (Breman and
Campbell, 1988). Hence, in Kenya 92% of symptomatic Pf infections with
RII-RIII parasitological responses became afebrile, although 78% of them only
resolved temporarily (Brandling-Bennett *et al.*, 1988). A certain level of immunity appears to be necessary as, in a Somalian study, the symptoms did not clear
as readily in the chloroquine-treated patients who were less immune (Warsame
et al., 1990).

The mode of action of chloroquine is still not agreed. However, digestion of
host-derived haemoglobin in the acid lysosome and alteration of lysosomal pH
appear to be important for the accumulation of chloroquine and its parasiti-
cidal action. Decreased chloroquine accumulation by increased drug efflux
(Krogstad *et al.*, 1987) is then a mechanism by which the parasite may decrease
its susceptibility to the drug. And indeed, resistance to chloroquine has been
reversed by partial blockage of the drug efflux by means of calcium channel
antagonists (Martin *et al.*, 1987). However, the reversal of resistance appears to
be possible also quite independently of calcium channels (Ye and van Dyke,
1988; Peters *et al.*, 1989). Multi-drug resistant genes (pF mdr_1, and pG mdr_2)
have been identified and considered as possibly involved in chloroquine
resistance (Foote *et al.*, 1989; Wilson *et al.*, 1989). Recently, however, there were
apparently conflicting findings in two studies trying to link *mdr* genes with
chloroquine resistance (Wellens *et al.*, 1990; Foote *et al.*, 1990). Clearly, more
genetic studies are needed to resolve this issue. Epidemiological studies on the
genetic variations may provide clues especially towards an understanding of the
apparently different ways resistance has evolved in different parts of the world.

Continuous or repeated drug pressure in animal models decreases the
susceptibilities of the different *Plasmodium* species to chloroquine and other
drugs (Peters, 1987). This situation does not necessarily apply to CRPf which
may not be induced but rather selected for by the drug. Haphazard chloroquine
use, often including use of subcurative doses on a wide scale, e.g. medicated salt
(Payne, 1988), has been postulated to have contributed greatly towards the
development of CRPf. However, in areas such as Liberia, despite intensive use of
chloroquine for many years, CRPf did not occur until resistant parasites were
imported (Björkman, 1985; Björkman *et al.*, 1991). However, once established,
CRPf appears to be intensified by drug pressure (Kremsner *et al.*, 1989) mainly
by selection for the resistant parasites in the human host (Brandling-Bennett *et
al.*, 1988; Warsame *et al.*, 1990) but also possibly by enhanced development in
mosquitoes feeding on infected blood containing residual chloroquine (Wilkinson *et al.*, 1976; Rosario *et al.*, 1988). In a recent report, this appeared not to be

valid for individual sublines of a *P. yoelii* strain, such as a chloroquine-resistant clone, although the enhancement was observed in the original strain (Ichimori *et al.*, 1990).

However, CRPf appears also to have developed and spread without undue drug pressure (Draper *et al.*, 1988). To explain this, the hypothesis has been the general biological advantage of resistant over sensitive parasites based on evidence from mouse models (Rosario *et al.*, 1978) and *in vitro* (Thaitong, 1983). Enhanced reproduction of CRPf in the mosquito has also been suggested for two anopheline species (Sucharit *et al.*, 1977). A general counter-argument to the hypothesis of genetic superiority of CRPf is to question why it did not evolve earlier and the resistant strains thus already outnumber the sensitive ones. A biological superiority of CRPf would imply continued high levels of resistance even after withdrawal of the drug, unless the resistance to chloroquine is associated with resistance of the alternative drugs. However, in a study from Thailand there were signs of gradual increase in Pf sensitivity to chloroquine between 1981 and 1986 possibly following the withdrawal of chloroquine as first-line treatment from 1972 (Thaitong *et al.*, 1988).

In an endemic area the two main means by which parasite growth and the parasite population are affected are chemotherapy and protective host immunity. As effects of chemotherapy and immunity are considered to be additive if not synergistic, individuals with low immunity were thought to be important for the propagation of CRPf. However, this cannot explain the fast propagation of CRPf in Africa, and the high herd immunity in most African countries would rather contradict the hypothesis.

Although high transmission and turnover of the parasite population in highly endemic areas of Africa combined with chloroquine use is important, another mechanism may also be suggested — a biological advantage of CRPf due to an antigenic difference of CRPf and thus relatively less protective immunity against such strains as compared with drug-sensitive ones. Recent epidemiological data from Tanzania supported the idea (Koella *et al.*, 1990). It would explain why in a highly endemic area CRPf gets quickly established and then remains at a fairly stable level and frequency. Individuals with low immunity are probably more important in the context of the manifestations of CRPf, as therapeutic failures in such people may increase the incidence of severe malaria. This can cause malaria 'outbreaks' both in fringe areas of malaria endemicity and in endemic areas where there are immigrants from non-endemic areas with low immunity (Figure 1).

Preconditions for the development and spread of drug resistance differ between the African and Asian continents. Migration of people carrying CRPf gametocytes has probably been of major importance for the spread of resistance between different endemic areas in Asia and Oceania, whereas on the African continent the spread has been a more steady flow. In the beginning there was a picture of a core area with high resistance and a peripheral area with parasites of

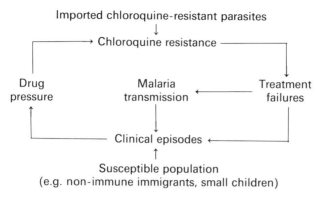

Figure 1   Increased malaria morbidity triggered by the development of chloroquine-resistant *Plasmodium falciparum*

low resistance, possibly consisting of hybrid resistant and sensitive forms. However, the parasites in Africa which have become resistant in the second half of the 1980s have rather shown an immediate development of a high level of resistance.

Sulfadoxine–pyrimethamine

Resistance to sulfadoxine–pyrimethamine (SP) has been reported mainly in areas of intense use, particularly Thailand and Kampuchea. By the mid-1970s treatment failures at the RIII level occurred in Thailand (Doberstyn *et al.*, 1976), and by 1980 drug failure rates were up to 90% (Pinichpongse *et al.*, 1982) and SP was largely replaced by quinine–tetracycline for clinical purposes. Resistance has lately also been reported from many other areas of South-East Asia and South America (Peters, 1987). Numerous sentinel cases of resistance to SP have also been reported from Africa in non-immune individuals, but generally clinical trials in semi-immunes have shown success rates between 85% and 100%. *In vitro* studies have confirmed the existence of isolates with resistance patterns but at a low frequency. West African studies have generally shown higher efficacy than East African studies. However, these studies have generally been performed before use of SP therapeutically on a large scale. Recent findings of significantly increased failure rate in individuals from Rwanda with low immunity, two years after introduction of the drug, are therefore quite alarming (Garcia Vidal *et al.*, 1989).

SP, being not too expensive (US$0.13 per treatment) and given conveniently as a single dose, today represents the first choice for treatment of clinical episodes of Pf malaria in Africa that are not life-threatening, but its efficacy needs to be closely monitored and increased resistance may be expected in the relatively near future.

Quinine

Quinine has remained the main therapeutic drug for CRPf malaria, although low sensitivity was reported in Brazil as early as 1910. Quinine has been used extensively in South-East Asia, where resistance to chloroquine and SP is especially high. The cure rates with quinine have now fallen substantially in some areas, even below 50% (Bunnag and Harinasuta, 1987; Giboda and Denis, 1988). Tetracycline has thus been added to provide higher cure rates. From other areas, including Africa, there are reports of sentinel cases of *in vivo* resistance, and *in vitro* studies in a few francophone countries in Africa have revealed reduced sensitivity. However, the significance of these findings remains unclear.

Chloroquine resistance has been suggested as a prerequisite for the development of quinine resistance in South-East Asia (Knowles *et al.*, 1984). The *in vitro* correlation between chloroquine resistance and reduced sensitivity to quinine in Africa (Liberia, Somalia, Cameroon), although not to the point of resistance (Brasseur *et al.*, 1988; Björkman *et al.*, 1991; Warsame *et al.*, 1991b), is therefore alarming as it may represent a first step towards further development of complete resistance on this continent.

Quinidine, the stereoisomer of quinine, has been found to be more active than quinine both in Asia (Sabchareon *et al.*, 1988) and Africa (Björkman *et al.*, 1991). However, it gives about two times lower blood concentration than quinine in equivalent doses and has higher cardiotropic affinity (Jamaludin *et al.*, 1988). In some African countries a combination of quinine, quinidine and chinonine (Quinimax) has been used for many years with possibly additive activity (Deloron *et al.*, 1989).

There are major compliance problems with quinine because of the regimen of two or three daily doses for seven days and the occurrence of side-effects. Only three days of quinine treatment may be needed for a clinical effect in symptomatic patients (Greenberg *et al.*, 1989) and even radical parasitological cure in semi-immune patients (Björkman *et al.*, 1991).

Mefloquine

Clinical trials of mefloquine conducted in the early 1980s in different areas of the world showed high efficacy (98–100%) (WHO, 1984) although in Thailand along the Kampuchean border the efficacy was only about 90% (WHO, personal communication). Field *in vitro* studies using standardized WHO microtests have mostly confirmed parasite susceptibilities of between 97% and 100% (Björkman and Phillips-Howard, 1990). In contrast, but with other methodologies and criteria for resistance, two recent studies have reported reduced susceptibility in several areas of West Africa (Oduola *et al.*, 1987; Simon *et al.*, 1988).

A general problem with mefloquine is the low therapeutic margin combined with high individual variations in concentrations of the active parent compound obtained. Hence, in contrast to the *in vivo* findings above, a high failure rate has recently been recorded in Malawian children below 5 years of age after a dose of 25 mg/kg, despite a profile of the *in vitro* tests which indicated sensitivity (Slutsker *et al.*, 1990). The failures were, however, strongly associated with low mefloquine concentrations, which were not necessarily due to vomiting.

Maybe the efficacy of mefloquine treatment is also largely dependent on the immune status; in a study from Burma (Tin *et al.*, 1982) semi-immune patients eventually cleared their parasitaemias despite transient blood films seven and 14 days after treatment.

The interpretation of *in vivo* and *in vitro* data with regard to mefloquine is obviously complex. More combined *in vivo* and *in vitro* studies in West Africa and other areas, preferably in individuals with low immunity, are necessary for a better understanding of the patterns of Pf susceptibility to mefloquine.

The modes of action of mefloquine and quinine are considered to be similar but *in vitro* studies from Thailand (Subsaeng *et al.*, 1986) have shown some cross-resistance. Similarly, epidemiological data from Thailand indicate partial cross-resistance between the two drugs. In Africa, some correlation of the drug susceptibility profiles was found in isolates from Cameroon (Brasseur *et al.*, 1988) and from Somalia (Warsame *et al.*, 1991b). However, with mefloquine and chloroquine, the picture is more obscure as *in vitro* data on cultured parasites (Knowles *et al.*, 1984) and wild isolates (Warsame *et al.*, 1991b) and the identification of potentially mefloquine-resistant parasites in West Africa indicate an inverse correlation between chloroquine and mefloquine resistance. In rodent malaria, however, both quinine and chloroquine resistance appear to enhance the development of mefloquine resistance (Peters, 1987) and the possibility that genuine use (in francophone West Africa) may indirectly have affected the susceptibility to mefloquine needs to be considered. No link of mefloquine resistance with *mdr* genes has yet been reported.

In conclusion, existing data tend to indicate that Pf parasites, potentially resistant to mefloquine treatment, may be found in different endemic areas before introduction of the drug. Considering this and the ease with which resistance can be induced in murine infections, a rapid evolution of drug resistance may be expected if mefloquine is used on a large scale in an endemic area.

Mefloquine–sulfadoxine–pyrimethamine

This triple combination (MSP), incorporating a reduced dose of mefloquine and thus having fewer mefloquine dose-dependent side-effects, has shown high activity and delayed development of resistance in animal models (Peters, 1987). Although some *in vitro* findings and one *in vivo* study have suggested antagonistic effects between the compounds, a recent *in vivo* study from Tanzania demonstrates an additive effect by use of this combination (Havemann, personal communication).

Clinical trials in the mid-1980s showed cure rates of 98–100% in Africa, South America and South-East Asia even though, in two of the areas, Brazil and Thailand, resistance to SP was already increasing (Peters, 1987). However, after its release in 1985 in Thailand, the efficacy dropped from 96% to below 50% in 1990 in two highly endemic areas (WHO, personal communication).

In human beings mefloquine has a longer half-life than sulfadoxine and pyrimethamine. Low non-inhibitory concentrations of mefloquine therefore persist in the blood for long periods, unprotected by the other drugs (White, 1987). The use of SP may thus prevent the development of mefloquine resistance in areas with low transmission but not in highly endemic areas where Pf is inoculated frequently.

The rapid development of resistance to MSP in the areas of Thailand where it was widely used suggests that the value of the combination may be limited in areas with an already high degree of SP resistance. A higher dose of mefloquine alone is probably a better choice in such conditions. The role of MSP in Africa where SP resistance is less pronounced remains uncertain and different aspects, such as costs, compliance, toxicity and efficacy of MSP, need to be compared with those for other drugs before a decision is taken.

Future prospects

From the US Army research programme screening for antimalarial activity one additional drug besides mefloquine has emerged: halofantrine. Both are unfortunately similar chemically and in their mode of action to quinine, and related development of resistance can therefore be expected and, indeed, has occurred in rodent malaria (Peters *et al.*, 1987). Different dose schedules are now being tested as the one-day course has provided only low cure rates in Thailand (WHO, personal communications).

More promising is the development of the sesquiterpenes, with the original compound, artemisinine, isolated from the old Chinese herbal remedy, qinghao. The presently developed analogues, artemether, arteether and sodium artesunate, have been shown to be very powerful schizonticides with apparently a low level of toxicity. Importantly, the mode of action appears to be different from that of existing antimalarial compounds. Development of resistance has been shown, however, as with all other antimalarial drugs, in rodent malaria (Chawira *et al.*, 1986). Preliminary data given from Thailand confirm the high clearance rates reported from China but with a tendency for recrudescence, which can probably be solved by increasing the length of treatment.

Another Chinese compound, pyronaridine, appears to be active against CRPf strains but shares structural similarities with amodiaquine, and results should be interpreted with caution (Peters, 1987). The toxicity issue also largely remains uncertain.

Another promising discovery, already mentioned, is the ability to reverse chloroquine resistance by use of verapamil (Martin et al., 1987) and several other compounds (Peters et al., 1989). These findings need to be confirmed in vivo, but toxicity issues with regard to the effect of accumulation of chloroquine also need to be addressed.

It must be concluded, however, that the scientific advances in development of new chemotherapeutic agents are very limited, reflecting both technical difficulties and great demands on resources. It is therefore understandable why the pharmaceutical industry has made only a limited commitment to the development of new antimalarial drugs.

General determinants of resistance

Resistance arises as a result of gene mutation and selection of resistant mutants (Beale, 1980). Laboratory and field data clearly indicate the effect of drug pressure on the selection of resistance in the parasite populations. This selection is thought to be enhanced by the use of subtherapeutic drug levels and by a flat dose–response curve to the drug (Peters, 1987) which would increase the number of surviving parasites. However, an opposite view has also been expressed after mathematical modelling indicating that higher doses may select more strongly for highly resistant parasites (Cross, 1987).

The conditions may vary with the type of drug and the *Plasmodium* species, as single exposure to a high concentration of pyrimethamine induces resistance in different Pf strains, whereas chloroquine resistance in animal models is more readily produced by treatment with low dosages that are gradually increased (Peters, 1987), indicating a series of mutations that may not even be induced in Pf malaria.

The role of immunity in propagating resistance is unclear but certainly immunity acts synergistically with chemotherapy and can enhance therapeutic effects and even parasite clearance of drug-resistant infections.

The bioavailability of a drug is an important parameter as there are large individual variations in pharmacokinetics. Different profiles of metabolism may create wide differences in activity; the main metabolite may be highly active (for proguanil) or inactive (for mefloquine). Finally, a long half-life enhances the development of drug resistance in endemic areas with high inoculation rates. This would imply a much higher tendency for resistance using mefloquine than quinine in sub-Saharan Africa.

Cross-resistance between drugs appears to be only partly resolved. There is a general tendency towards multiple resistance to the existing antimalarial drugs, and chloroquine resistance appears to be associated with decreased quinine but not necessarily mefloquine susceptibility.

Implications for malaria control

There is little information on the specific impact of CRPf on the health of the affected population. It is, however, clear that clinical malaria episodes will increase in frequency and possibly severity because of unsuccessful treatment or chemoprophylaxis and increased transmission of Pf malaria (Figure 1).

A major problem is that chloroquine can no longer be trusted when used for treatment after presumptive diagnosis. Whereas previously a persisting fever after the chloroquine treatment indicated an aetiology other than malaria, today this may also be due to an unsuccessfully treated Pf infection, which may become even more severe. This situation clearly enhances the need for proper parasite diagnosis and referral.

Great efforts have been made to contain the development of drug resistance. Primaquine which is gametocyticidal has been added to chloroquine for presumptive treatment although on theoretical grounds this policy may favour the spread of CRPf in highly endemic areas. Vector control measures need to be considered in selected situations, although in India they have had little impact in containing CRPf. The use of combinations of drugs has not been tried systematically, although MSP had only limited value in Thailand, where SP resistance was already highly developed.

The relative costs in US dollars of the existing antimalarials per treatment episode for an adult have recently been calculated as: 0.08 for chloroquine, 0.13 for SP, 0.99 for quinine i.v. and 1.50 for quinine p.o., 1.92 for mefloquine, and 5.31 for halofantrine (WHO, 1990). These calculations indicate that apart from SP the alternatives to chloroquine represent substantial increases in therapeutic costs.

Self-treatment with chloroquine will thus continue to be attempted first at the time of fever episode; in rural Africa about 50% of infected individuals are believed to utilize health centres when they have malaria-like symptoms (Deming *et al.*, 1989). This utilization clearly depends in part on the distance from such health centres (Rooth *et al.*, 1991).

At the health clinic a decision to give chloroquine will depend on a patient's clinical presentation, the expected level of immunity, possible previous treatment, the resistance pattern in the area, the cost, availability and toxicity of alternative drugs and the possibility of referral of the patient. In Africa, considering costs and the present situation with regard to drug resistance, chloroquine and to some extent SP will remain the standard antimalarials for at least the near future. Many clinical episodes treated with chloroquine will therefore only resolve temporarily. This obviously is a more complex situation than before the advent of chloroquine resistance and therefore demands a reconsideration of malaria control strategies at primary health care level and necessitates retraining of health workers at peripheral as well as more central levels.

A practical question is when to switch to an alternative drug. Persisting parasites on the fourth day after treatment (Schapira *et al.*, 1988) and persistent or recurrent fever may be suggested as an indication, but depend on facilities for microscopy. It was recorded in a Tanzanian village that, of children still sick after treatment at the rural health clinic, 37% would go back to the clinic, 39% would visit the traditional healer and 24% would not seek any further medical assistance (Rooth *et al.*, 1991). That only about one-third would return for alternative medical treatment is clearly alarming in the context of the frequent resistance and thus failure of the first-line drug chloroquine in Africa.

The necessity to restrict drug use is obvious although some degree of over-prescription is inevitable. Optimally no antimalarial treatment should be given without a microscopically confirmed malaria diagnosis. This policy is clearly not possible in all instances. However, it may be realistic to link the deployment of second- and third-line drugs to microscopical diagnosis. Here again, an improvement of health care capacity including training in microscopy is an important target for improved malaria control.

Chemoprophylaxis during pregnancy is another issue that needs to be addressed in the context of CRPf. A decreased efficacy of chloroquine and an uncertainty about compliance may influence some authorities to be nihilistic about chemoprophylaxis. However, the benefits for the mother and the fetus of preventing malaria during pregnancy must be considered in relation to efficacy, compliance, costs and possible side-effects not only of chloroquine but also of mefloquine and proguanil, the latter possibly combined with a short-acting sulpha drug.

National monitoring systems of drug efficacy are necessary for continuous adjustment of treatment policies. These should primarily be based on standardized *in vivo* evaluation of clearance of symptoms and parasitaemias by the antimalarial drugs that are of operational interest. *In vitro* testing of the susceptibility of Pf isolates to the drugs indicates the resistance profile of the parasite population, but requires sophisticated methodology. Also it does not account for the immune status and pharmacokinetic profile in the human population and may thus not always reflect the clinical and parasitological effect of the drug in that population.

Prompt recognition of probable malaria infection followed by efficacious treatment is the key to prevention of malaria morbidity and mortality. Drug resistance has made this goal more difficult. Improved health care must be linked to improved community education. Parents and communities must be more involved in the process of disease recognition, therapy and prevention. A better understanding is needed of people's perception of malaria illness and health-seeking behaviour, which may and should vary substantially depending on endemicity.

References

Allen SJ, Otoo LN, Cooke GA, O'Donnell A and Greenwood BM (1990) Sensitivity of *Plasmodium falciparum* to chlorproguanil in Gambian children after five years of continuous chemoprophylaxis. *Transactions of the Royal Society of Tropical Medicine and Hygiene, 84,* 218

Beale GH (1980) The genetics of drug resistance in malaria parasites. *Bulletin of the World Health Organization, 58,* 799–804

Björkman A (1985) Malaria epidemiology, drug protection and drug susceptibility in a holoendemic area of Liberia. Thesis, Karolinska Institute

Björkman A, Brohult I, Willcox M, Pehrson PO, Rombo L, Hedman P, Hetland G, Kollie E, Hanson AP and Bengtsson E (1985a). Malaria control by chlorproguanil. I. Clinical effects and *Plasmodium falciparum in vivo* susceptibility maintained after seven years of monthly drug administration to the children in a Liberian village. *Annals of Tropical Medicine and Parasitology, 79,* 597–601

Björkman A, Rombo L, Hetland G, Willcox M and Hanson AP (1985b) Susceptibility of *Plasmodium falciparum* to chloroquine in northern Liberia after 20 years of chemosuppression and therapy. *Annals of Tropical Medicine and Parasitology, 79,* 603–606

Björkman A and Phillips-Howard PA (1990) The epidemiology of drug-resistant malaria. *Transactions of the Royal Society of Tropical Medicine and Hygiene, 84,* 177–180

Björkman A and Phillips-Howard PA (1991) Adverse drug reactions to sulfa drugs: implications for malaria chemotherapy. *Bulletin of the World Health Organization, 69,* 297–304

Björkman A, Willcox M, Marbiah N and Payne D (1991) Susceptibility of *P. falciparum* to different doses of quinine *in vivo* and *in vitro* and to quinidine in relation to chloroquine in Liberia. *Bulletin of the World Health Organization 69,* 459–465

Brandling-Bennett AD, Oloo AJ, Watkins WM, Boriga DA, Kariuki DM and Collins WE (1988) Chloroquine treatment of falciparum malaria in an area of Kenya of intermediate chloroquine resistance. *Transactions of the Royal Society of Tropical Medicine and Hygiene, 82,* 833–837

Brasseur P, Kouamouo I, Brandicourt O, Mayaou-Somo R and Druilhe P (1988) Patterns of *in vitro* resistance to chloroquine, quinine and mefloquine of *Plasmodium falciparum* in Cameroon, 1985–1986. *American Journal of Tropical Medicine and Hygiene, 39,* 166–172

Breman IG and Campbell CC (1988) Combating severe malaria in African children. *Bulletin of the World Health Organization, 66,* 611–620

Bunnag D and Harinasuta T (1987) Quinine and quinidine in malaria in Thailand. *Acta Leidensia, 55,* 163–166

Chawira AN, Warhurst DC and Peters W (1986) Qinghaosu resistance in rodent malaria. *Transactions of the Royal Society of Tropical Medicine and Hygiene, 86,* 477–480

Clyde DF (1967) *Malaria in Tanzania.* Oxford University Press, London

Cross AP (1987) A computer simulation model for the development of drug resistance by *Plasmodium falciparum.* PhD thesis, Yale University, New Haven

Deloron P, Lepers IP, Verdier F, Chougnet C, Remanamirija IA, Andriangatianarason MD, Coulanges P and Jaureguiberry G (1989) Efficacy of a 3-day oral regimen of a quinine–quinidine–cinchonine association (Quinimax) for treatment of falciparum malaria in Madagascar. *Transactions of the Royal Society of Tropical Medicine and Hygiene, 83,* 751–754

Deming MS, Gayibor A, Murphy K, Jones TS and Kaisa T (1989) Home treatment of febrile children with antimalarial drugs in Togo. *Bulletin of the World Health Organization, 67,* 695–700

Doberstyn EB, Hall AP, Vetvutanapibul K and Sonkom P (1976) Single dose therapy of falciparum malaria using pyrimethamine in combination with diformyldapsone or sulfadoxine. *American Journal of Tropical Medicine and Hygiene, 25,* 14–19

Draper CC, Hills M, Kilimali AEB and Brubaker G (1988) Serial studies on the evolution of drug resistance in malaria in an area of East Africa: findings from 1979 up to 1986. *Journal of Tropical Medicine and Hygiene, 91,* 265–273

Foote SJ, Thompson JK, Cowman AF and Kemp DJ (1989) Amplification of the multidrug resistance gene in some chloroquine-resistant isolates of *P. falciparum. Cell, 57,* 921–930

Foote SJ, Galatis D and Cowman AF (1990a) Amino acids in the dihydrofolate reductase thymidylate synthase gene of *Plasmodium falciparum* involved in cycloguanil tance differ from those involved in pyrimethamine resistance. *Proceedings of the National Academy of Sciences USA, 87,* 3014–3017.

Foote SJ, Kyle DE, Martin RK, Oduola AMJ, Forsyth K, Kemp DJ and Cowman AF (1990b) Several alleles of the multidrug resistance gene are closely linked to chloroquine resistance in *Plasmodium falciparum. Nature, 345,* 255–258

Garcia-Vidal J, Ngirabega JD, Soldevila M, Navarro R and Bada JL (1989) Evolution of resistance of *Plasmodium falciparum* to antimalarial drugs in Rwanda 1985–1987. *Transactions of the Royal Society of Tropical Medicine and Hygiene, 83,* 490

Giboda M and Denis MB (1988) Response of Kampuchean strains of *Plasmodium falciparum* to antimalarials in *in vivo* assessment of quinine and quinine plus tetracycline: multiple drug resistance *in vivo. Journal of Tropical Medicine and Hygiene, 91,* 205–211

Greenberg AE, Nguyen-Dinh P, Davachi F, Yemvula B, Malanda N, Nzeza M, Williams SB, De Zwart JF and Zneza M, (1989) Intravenous quinine therapy of hospitalized children with *Plasmodium falciparum* malaria in Kinshasa, Zaire. *American Journal of Tropical Medicine and Hygiene, 40,* 360–364

Havemann K, Kihamia CM, Gallachi A, Lebbad M, Bengquist Y and Bjorkman A (1991) Additive activity of mefloquine and sulfadoxine/pyrimethamine against *Plasmodium falciparum* in Tanzania (submitted for publication)

Ichimori K, Curtis CF and Targett GAT (1990) The effects of chloroquine on the infectivity of chloroquine-sensitive and -resistant populations of *Plasmodium yoelii nigeriensis* to mosquitoes. *Parasitology, 100,* 377–381

Jamaludin A, Mohamed M, Navaratnam V, Mohamed N, Yeoh E and Wernsdorfer W (1988) Single-dose comparative kinetics and bioavailability study of quinine hydrochloride, quinidine sulfate and quinidine bisulfate sustained-release in healthy male volunteers. *Acta Leidensia, 57,* 39–46

Karwacki JJ, Shanks GD, Limsomwong N and Singharaj P (1990) Proguanil sulphonamide for malaria prophylaxis. *Transactions of the Royal Society of Tropical Medicine and Hygiene, 84,* 55–57

Keuter M, Van Eijk A, Hoogstrate M, Raasveld M, Van de Ree M, Ngwawe WA, Watkins WM, Were IBO and Brandling-Bennett AD (1990) Comparison of chloroquine, pyrimethamine and sulfadoxine, and chlorproguanil and dapsone as treatment for falciparum malaria in pregnant and non-pregnant women, Kahamega district, Kenya. *British Medical Journal, 1301,* 466–470

Knowles G, Davidson WE, Jolley D and Alpers MP (1984) The relationship between the *in vitro* response of *Plasmodium falciparum* to chloroquine, quinine and mefloquine. *Transactions of the Royal Society of Tropical Medicine and Hygiene, 78,* 146–150

Koella JC, Hatz C, Mshinda H, de Savigny D, Macpherson CNL, Degrémont AA and

Tanner M (1990) *In vitro* resistance patterns of *Plasmodium falciparum* to chloroquine: a reflection of strain-specific immunity? *Transactions of the Royal Society of Tropical Medicine and Hygiene, 84,* 662–665

Kouznetsov BL, Storey I, Kilama W and Payne D (1980) Spread of pyrimethamine-resistant strains of *Plasmodium falciparum* into new areas of North-East Tanzania with absence of drug pressure. *WHO MAL/80.926*

Kremsner PG, Zotter GM, Feldmeier GH, Graninger W, Kollaritsch M, Wiedermann G, Rocha RM and Wernsdorfer W (1989) *In vitro* drug sensitivity of *Plasmodium falciparum* in Acre, Brazil. *Bulletin of the World Health Organization, 67,* 289–293

Krogstad DJ, Gluzman IY, Kyle DE, Oduola AMJ, Martin SK, Milhous WK and Schleringer PH (1987) Efflux of chloroquine from *Plasmodium falciparum*: mechanism of chloroquine resistance. *Science, 238,* 1283–1285

Limsomwong N, Pange LW and Singharaj P (1988) Malaria prophylaxis with proguanil in children living in a malaria endemic area. *American Journal of Tropical Medicine and Hygiene, 38,* 231–236

Martin KS, Oduola AMI and Milhous WK (1987) Reversal of chloroquine resistance in *Plasmodium falciparum* by verapamil. *Science, 235,* 899–902

Oduola AM, Milhous WK, Salako LA, Walker O and Desjardins RE (1987) Reduced *in vitro* susceptibility to mefloquine in West African isolates of *Plasmodium falciparum*. *Lancet, ii,* 572–573

Pang LW, Limsomwong N, Singharaj P and Canfield CI (1989) Malaria prophylaxis with proguanil and sulfadoxazole in children living in a malaria endemic area. *Bulletin of the World Health Organization, 67,* 51–58

Payne D (1988) Did medicated salt hasten the spread of chloroquine resistance in *Plasmodium falciparum*? *Parasitology Today, 4,* 112–115

Peters W (1987) *Chemotherapy and Drug Resistance in Malaria.* Academic Press, London

Peters W, Robinson BL and Ellis DS (1987) The chemotherapy of rodent malaria. XLII. Halofantrine and halofantrine resistance. *Annals of Tropical Medicine and Parasitology, 81,* 639–646

Peters W, Ekong R, Robinson BL, Warhurst DC and Panx Q (1989) Antihistaminic drugs that reverse chloroquine resistance in *Plasmodium falciparum*. *Lancet, ii,* 334–335

Peterson DS, Milhous WK and Wellems TE (1990) Molecular basis of differential resistance to cycloguanil and pyrimethamine in *Plasmodium falciparum* malaria. *Proceedings of the National Academy of Sciences USA, 87,* 3018–3022

Phillips-Howard PA, Radalowicz A, Mitchel J and Bradley DJ (1990) Risk of malaria in British residents returning from malarious areas. *British Medical Journal, 300,* 499–503

Rooth I, Johansson M, Phillips-Howard PA, Nilsson B and Bjorkman A (1991) Perceptions and health seeking behaviour related to holoendemic malaria in two Tanzanian villages with different access to health care. (Submitted for publication)

Rosario VE, Hall R, Walliker D and Beale GH (1978) Persistence of drug resistant malaria parasites. *Lancet, i,* 185–187

Rosario V, Vaughan V, Murphy M, Harrod V and Coleman R (1988) The effect of chloroquine on the sporogonic cycle of *Plasmodium falciparum* and *Plasmodium berghei* in anopheline mosquitoes. *Acta Leidensia, 57,* 53–60

Sabchareon A, Chongsuphajaisiddhi T, Sinhasivanon V, Chanthavanich P and Attanath P (1988) *In vivo* and *in vitro* responses to quinine and quinidine of *Plasmodium falciparum*. *Bulletin of the World Health Organization, 66,* 347–352

Schapira A, Almeida Franco LT, Averkiev L, Omawale, Schwalbach J and Suleimanov G (1988) The *Plasmodium falciparum* chloroquine *in vivo* test: extended follow up is more important than parasite counting. *Transactions of the Royal Society of Tropical Medicine and Hygiene, 82,* 39–43

Simon F, Le-Bras J, Gaudebout C and Girard PM (1988) Reduced sensitivity of *Plasmodium falciparum* to mefloquine in West Africa. *Lancet, i*, 467–468

Slutsker LM, Khoromana CO, Payne D, Allen CR, Wirima JJ, Heymann DL, Patchen L and Steketee RW (1990) Mefloquine therapy for *Plasmodium falciparum* malaria in children under 5 years of age in Malawi: *in vivo/in vitro* efficacy and correlation of drug concentration with parasitological outcome. *Bulletin of the World Health Organization, 68*, 53–59

Subsaeng L, Wernsdorfer WH, Rooney W (1986) Sensitivity to quinine and mefloquine of *Plasmodium falciparum* in Thailand. *Bulletin of the World Health Organization, 64*, 759–765

Sucharit S, Surathin K, Tumrasvin W and Sucharit P (1977) Chloroquine resistant *Plasmodium falciparum* in Thailand: susceptibility of *Anopheles*. *Journal of the Medical Association of Thailand, 60*, 648–654

Thaitong S (1983) Clones of different sensitivities in drug resistant isolates of *Plasmodium falciparum*. *Bulletin of the World Health Organization, 79*, 37–41

Thaitong S, Suebsaeng L, Rooney W and Beale GH (1988) Evidence of increased chloroquine sensitivity in Thai isolates of *Plasmodium falciparum*. *Transactions of the Royal Society of Tropical Medicine and Hygiene, 82*, 37–38

Tin F, Hlaing N and Lasserre R (1982). Single-dose treatment of falciparum malaria with mefloquine: field studies with different doses in semi-immune adults and children in Burma. *Bulletin of the World Health Organization, 60*, 913–917

Ward SA, Watkins WM, Mberu E, Saunders JE, Koech DK, Gilles HM, Howells RE and Breckenridge AM (1989) Inter-subject variability in the metabolism of proguanil to the active metabolite cycloguanil in man. *British Journal of Clinical Pharmacology, 27*, 781–787

Warsame M, Wernsdorfer W, Eriksson O and Bjorkman A (1990) Isolated malaria outbreak in Somalia: role of chloroquine resistant *Plasmodium falciparum* demonstrated in Balcad epidemic. *Journal of Tropical Medicine and Hygiene, 93*, 284–289

Warsame M, Wernsdorfer WH, Willcox M, Kulane AA and Bjorkman A (1991a) The changing pattern of *Plasmodium falciparum* susceptibility to chloroquine but not to mefloquine in a mesoendemic area of Somalia. *Transactions of the Royal Society of Tropical Medicine and Hygiene 85*, 200–203

Warsame M, Wernsdorfer WH, Payne D and Bjorkman A (1991b) *In vitro* susceptibility of *Plasmodium falciparum* to chloroquine, mefloquine, quinine and sulfadoxine/pyrimethamine in Somalia: relationships between the responses to the different drugs. *Transactions of the Royal Society of Tropical Medicine and Hygiene*, (in press)

Watkins WM, Howells RE, Brandling-Bennett AD and Koech DK (1987) *In vitro* susceptibility of *Plasmodium falciparum* isolates from Jilore, Kenya, to antimalarial drugs. *American Journal of Tropical Medicine and Hygiene, 37*, 445–451

Watkins WM, Brandling-Bennett AD, Nevill CG, Carter JY, Boriga DA, Howells RE and Koech DK (1988) Chlorproguanil/dapsone for the treatment of non-severe *Plasmodium falciparum* malaria in Kenya: a pilot study. *Transactions of the Royal Society of Tropical Medicine and Hygiene, 82*, 398–403

Wellems TE, Panton LJ, Gluzman IY, de Rosario VE, Gwadz RW, Walker Jonah A and Krogstad DJ (1990) Chloroquine resistance not linked to mdr-like genes in a *Plasmodium falciparum* cross. *Nature, 345*, 253–255

White NJ (1987) Combination treatment for falciparum prophylaxis. *Lancet, i*, 680–681

WHO (1984) *Advances in Malaria Chemotherapy*. World Health Organization, Geneva, Technical Report Series no. 711

WHO (1990) *Practical chemotherapy of malaria*. World Health Organization, Geneva, Technical Report Series no. 805

Wilkinson RN, Noeypatimanondh S and Gould DJ (1976) Infectivity of falciparum malaria patients for anopheline mosquitoes before and after chloroquine treatment. *Transactions of the Royal Society of Tropical Medicine and Hygiene*, 70, 306–307

Wilson CM, Serrano AE, Wasley A, Bogenschutz MP, Shankar AH and Wirth DF (1989) Amplification of a gene related to mammalian mdr genes in drug-resistant *Plasmodium falciparum*. *Science*, 244, 1184–1186

Ye ZG and Van Dyke K (1988) Reversal of chloroquine resistance in falciparum malaria independent of calcium channels. *Biochemical and Biophysical Research Communications*, 155, 476–481

WORKSHOP REPORT AND RECOMMENDATIONS
RAPPORTEUR: NICHOLAS J. WHITE

Resistance in *Plasmodium falciparum* has developed to all currently available antimalarial drugs. The prospects for the future are bleak as there is little pharmaceutical industry interest in antimalarial drug development, and there are very few new drugs on the near horizon.

Emergence of resistance

Resistance to chloroquine and pyrimethamine is widespread, but sulfadoxine-pyrimethamine remains a first-line treatment in areas with recent chloroquine resistance. The role of the antimalarial biguanides in both prophylaxis and treatment (where they should be combined with sulphones or sulphonamides) needs to be defined, as resistance develops more slowly in this class of compounds. In this context the mechanisms underlying the emergence of antimalarial drug resistance need to be characterized. The notion that drugs such as pyrimethamine, sulfadoxine or mefloquine which are eliminated slowly are more likely to encourage the development of resistance than more rapidly eliminated drugs (quinine, biguanides, artemesinine derivatives) needs to be investigated. Patients treated with slowly eliminated drugs return to malaria transmission areas with subtherapeutic blood concentrations of the antimalarial drugs that persist for weeks or months. The exact duration of therapy for short half-life drugs needs to be defined in patient groups of different ages and levels of background immunity. Patient acceptability and compliance are major factors determining therapeutic outcome.

Evaluation of antimalarial drug efficacy

Chloroquine is still a very useful drug but resistance continues to increase in *P. falciparum*, and may now be emerging in *P. vivax* in eastern Asia. Deployment of chloroquine (and, indeed, any of the antimalarial drugs) should be based on operational definitions of resistance derived from short-term (within one week) and long-term (one month) post-treatment *clinical* assessments. The parasitological response, i.e. the conventional *in vivo* assessment and, to a lesser degree, the *in vitro* drug sensitivity tests provide complementary information but should not be primary determinants of treatment policies. Obviously the significance of positive blood smears following treatment will depend very much on the immune status of the patient, and the criteria for re-treatment or changes in antimalarial therapy *recommendations* must depend on local patterns of response. We recommend that sentinel posts should be set up at different places within malarious countries for such clinical antimalarial drug monitoring. This monitoring will allow regional decisions to be made on the basis of local patterns of therapeutic response (i.e. drug sensitivity and immunity). These posts should report to central government. A team to provide confirmatory parasitological and, if necessary, *in vitro* testing should go to posts reporting poor therapeutic responses in order to investigate and verify the local pattern of drug sensitivity. Guidelines should be drawn up locally providing criteria on which a decision to change treatment recommendations should be made, and giving advice on the treatment of drug failures. Alternative therapy should be made available. This structure of continuous monitoring should be supported, and advice on data interpretation and decision making should be provided, by international bodies such as the World Health Organization.

Control of drugs

The registration of effective drugs which are not yet needed in a country should be delayed until the onset of resistance. Drugs of potential value for severe malaria (notably the artemesinine derivatives) should not be made available as oral formulations for uncomplicated malaria unless there are no effective alternatives. This policy, it is hoped, will delay the onset of resistance.

Pharmacological research

Further investigations on approaches to prolong the 'usefulness' of chloroquine, e.g. reversal of resistance, should be pursued.

Antimalarial drug use in the community

More information is needed on health-seeking behaviour and the use of traditional remedies and antimalarial drugs in the community.

Governments and international organizations should be encouraged to provide incentives to commercial pharmaceutical companies to develop new antimalarial drugs. The passage of drugs from the bench to clinical testing, and their course through the maze of drug regulatory requirements, should be facilitated.

The distribution and use of antimalarial drugs—not a pretty picture

Susan D.F. Foster

London School of Hygiene and Tropical Medicine, UK

Introduction

WHO estimates show that 40 % of the world's population is exposed to malaria (WHO, 1990). The same report noted that 'the situation in the world as a whole is far from improving'. The goal of world-wide eradication has been abandoned, for the time being at least; yet vestiges of eradication-oriented policies persist, often to the detriment of realistic control efforts. Malaria chemotherapy seems to be a good example of the old adage, 'the best is the enemy of the good'.

Another WHO report entitled *The World Drug Situation* estimates that as many as 2500 million people have no access to basic, essential drugs (WHO, 1988). Of course, many (if not most) of these people are the same ones who are exposed to malaria. Most of the developing countries spend less than US$5 per person annually on drugs, and resource constraints for malaria treatment and control are severe, and getting worse. The most notable change as far as malaria treatment is concerned is the increasing tendency towards self-medication for malaria. Only recently has this been recognized, in part owing to the unstinting efforts of anthropologists and social scientists to document the way drugs are really used. In this paper I shall review the evidence regarding the conditions in which antimalarials are distributed and used in developing countries, with emphasis on the unofficial, illicit distribution channels and on self-medication, which (whether we like it or not) now characterizes most antimalarial use in the developing world.

The distribution of antimalarials

In most countries there are typically four main distribution and supply networks for antimalarial drugs. These were described by the WHO (1990) as follows:

(1) *The public sector* includes the ministry of health facilities, the national teaching hospital, the national malaria control programme, the social security institute, and the military and police, etc. Typically these are funded

out of government revenues; in addition, the population is often asked to pay a 'user fee' at the time of consultation.

(2) *The private non-profit sector* is usually made up primarily of mission hospitals and other non-governmental services. This sector often receives some financial support from the government, as well as from user charges and external support from non-governmental organizations and churches.

(3) *The private commercial sector* is composed of private physicians, hospitals and clinics, private drug importers and pharmacies, and other outlets such as general stores and drug depots which are licensed to sell a limited range of drugs. It is usually self-financing although there may be significant subsidies from the government in the form of direct payments, tax concessions, preferential access to undervalued foreign exchange, or tariff protection from imports.

(4) *The private 'unofficial' or 'informal' sector* is composed of unofficial sales points such as market and street sellers, distributors of pilfered, counterfeit or adulterated drugs, etc. Despite the illegality of such practices in most countries, these activities are usually tolerated and those who carry them out may be well integrated into the local community. Such distribution in many countries accounts for a significant portion of the antimalarial drugs consumed. This sector is financed by sales revenues (and indirectly by public revenues where pilferage from government facilities is widespread).

The use of antimalarials within the context of malaria control programmes is well documented, especially in Asia (Somkid, 1983; Mills, 1990), but there is less information about the distribution through the official routine public health channels. In general, however, when the drugs are allocated to different health facilities, there are many competing demands. Specialists at the central hospital are geographically closer, and politically more powerful than remote health workers. As a result they get priority over rural health centres and hospitals in the allocation of available drugs. Drugs tend to 'stick' at central level when there is an overall shortage.

Even less is known about the very significant part of antimalarials distributed through unofficial channels and the private sector. Within the private sector, it is difficult to know what percentage is sold through 'official' pharmacies and what percentage is sold by rural stores and street sellers, since many of these purchase their drugs at official pharmacies. At lower levels of the 'unofficial' distribution system, a reduced range of antimalarials is available, usually chloroquine, and occasionally amodiaquine and sulfadoxine–pyrimethamine. It appears therefore that on average about half of the antimalarial drugs are distributed through the public sector including through national malaria control programmes, which account for 25–30% of the total. It can then be inferred that about half is distributed through the private sector.

The number of 'official ethical pharmacies' supplying the private sector is of course limited by the number of pharmacists available to staff them, and in many countries there are simply not enough pharmacists to staff more than a handful of pharmacies. These are usually in urban areas, especially in the capital city. As a result 'unofficial' outlets of various types typically account for as much as 25% of the total of drugs distributed; in some countries the percentage may be significantly higher and in rural areas they may account for most of the drugs distributed. The non-governmental organizations and mission facilities also account for a considerable portion in many countries. In Kenya, for example, they account for about 35% of drugs distributed. Therefore, the approximate breakdown for distribution to the consumer of antimalarials may be as described in Table 1.

Self-medication for malaria

Evidence from several countries indicates that self-medication may account for as much as half of all consumption, especially in rural areas. Reports from various countries show that general stores or market sellers may sell as much or possibly more chloroquine than is distributed through the health services. In Pikine, a suburb of Dakar, Senegal, for example, private street-traders sell drugs valued at 32 million CFA francs (US$125 000) whereas the government provides only 3 million CFA francs-worth; local self-financing schemes provide a further 40 million CFA francs. Such 'illicit' sellers therefore account for some 43% by value of drugs sold. In Pikine, street sellers have differentiated the antimalarial drugs market into those for 'prophylaxis' and those for 'cure'; the latter are up to ten times more expensive. Typically they provide chloroquine at 5 CFA francs per tablet (100 mg base) for weekly *prevention*, in a dose of two tablets once a week. For *treatment*, however, they propose amodiaquine (200 mg) at 25 CFA francs per tablet, two to four tablets to be taken at once (Fassin, 1988). These sellers, mostly recent immigrants to Dakar from rural

Table 1   Estimated percentage of antimalarial drugs distributed by channel

Sector	% of total
Public sector	**40–60**
National malaria control programmes	20–30
Primary health care and hospital use	20–30
Private sector[a]	**40–60**
'Official' ethical pharmacies	20–40
'Unofficial' outlets and sellers	20–50
Non-governmental organizations and clinics	25–40

[a] Private sector totals add to more than 100% since 'unofficial' outlets are often supplied through 'official' pharmacies.
Source: author's estimates.

areas, are highly organized and belong to a Moslem brotherhood (the *Mourides*) which supplies their drugs and protects them, and intervenes in cases of difficulties with the law (Fassin, 1986).

Similarly, in 1983 in rural Zimbabwe (before the introduction of the Zimbabwe Essential Drugs Programme) rural shopkeepers accounted for 43% of the consumption of chloroquine in the local area; whereas rural health facilities gave away free about 56%. Reasons people gave for patronizing the stores included the lack of queues, the convenient late hours of the stores, a suspicion of 'free' things, including drugs, their dislike of being asked questions or being physically examined, and the generally more friendly and helpful attitude of the shopkeepers (Raynal, 1985). In Saradidi, Kenya, before the initiation of a control programme, 53% of people in the area bought antimalarials from shops; the reasons given were that other sources were too far away, the shops were open in emergencies, the hospital or dispensary had no drugs, they had good past experience with the shops, and the shopkeeper gave advice, especially on dosage. But following the establishment of a community-based programme using village health volunteers to distribute chloroquine, shop use declined significantly (Mburu *et al.*, 1987). And in Mara, Tanzania, 72% of people got chloroquine from sources other than the official chemoprophylaxis programme; these included official sources such as the maternal and child health (MCH) clinic (55%), the dispensary (98%), and the hospital (18%); and unofficial outlets including shops (41%) and the market (10%) (MacCormack and Lwihula, 1983).

In Togo 83% of children with fever had been treated at home with chloroquine. Two-thirds of the mothers had obtained the drug from private sellers, who would sell chloroquine (100 mg base) at 10 CFA francs per tablet (about US$0.04). For two to six tablets they would give a discount, bringing the price to just over 8 CFA francs per tablet. There was at least one full-time vendor of chloroquine in 11 of the 13 sites studied (Deming *et al.*, 1989).

People often have stocks of drugs in their homes; Haak found in Brazil that many homes had various drugs, some of which had been prescribed by a physician; many were past the expiry date and had deteriorated (Haak, 1988). In Tanzania people liked to keep a reserve of antimalarials; one of the reasons given for the failure of a malaria prophylaxis programme was that the chloroquine intended for prophylaxis of the children was viewed by adults as 'a resource to be shared by all with fever, not necessarily the sole prerogative of well young children' (MacCormack and Lwihula, 1983). Drug trials involving use of placebos must take account of the fact that people tend to save drugs for future illnesses; in particular, the introduction of placebo antimalarials into the pool of drugs which may be used for self-medication poses risks which should be taken into account in design of the trials.

Why does a family make a decision to self-medicate? When a person in a family has a fever, especially a child, a decision has to be made quickly. The mother knows only that the child has fever and that malaria is common; she has to decide, on the basis of inadequate information, common sense, and the local beliefs about health and disease, what course of action to take. She also has to take account of the options open to her as far as distance to travel, cash required, etc. Not surprisingly, in many areas where malaria is endemic the mother takes the risk that the situation will resolve itself and treats the child herself, or with local resources. This will probably mean self-medication with drugs already in the home or with drugs purchased locally on the market. Only when she sees that home treatment is not working will she consider taking the child for professional care. At this point she has to organize care for the other children, obtain the cash needed, etc.; it may take a day or more to organize the trip to the health facility. Given the time already spent waiting to see the effect of the self-medication, a two-day delay in seeking care would not be unusual.

This anecdote gives some indication why self-medication is so widespread. The reasons fall into three main categories: inappropriate or unrealistic malaria treatment policies or drug regulations; poor quality or inconvenience of the health services; and lack of money or other economic barriers to seeking care. These, as well as some of the consequences, are examined more fully below.

Inappropriate policies

Ironically, people may be forced by the health services to resort to self-medication. Malaria treatment policy in some countries dates from the 'eradication days', and has not kept pace with changes in the resources available and the general situation. A WHO working group referred to a situation in which the malaria services 'may be frankly counterproductive (where they have become bureaucracies preoccupied with self-preservation)... In many countries... these systems persist, with attention to diagnosis and treatment remaining secondary to grander but possibly unrealistic objectives' (WHO, 1990). An example of such a policy occurred in the Philippines, where a malaria treatment policy geared to 'best practice' and requiring microscopic diagnosis had become impractical owing to changes in resource allocation for malaria. This failure had two serious consequences: it undermined the position of primary health care outreach workers, and it forced people to self-medicate. How did this happen? The policy was to treat only upon confirmation of a positive blood slide. In remote rural areas, however, this meant people had to travel far to reach the clinic for a slide to be taken; but the slide could only be read by microscopists some hours distant, and whose role had been expanded from the original one of malaria microscopy alone to general laboratory microscopy. The result was that as much as six weeks could elapse between the first visit and confirmation of the positive smear. Clearly people could not wait six weeks for treatment; only 10% even returned for the results of their smear, and most resorted to self-medication with a few tablets of sulfadoxine–pyrimethamine purchased in the local shop.

Meanwhile, the primary health care nurse–midwife, who was under instructions to treat only confirmed cases of malaria, was obliged to countermand her orders and provide presumptive treatment on the basis of her clinical diagnosis in order to maintain her credibility with the population. When slide results were available, it turned out that she was correct in 92 % of cases (Gomes and Salazar, 1990). Clearly, a change in policy is called for.

The Philippines situation also illustrates another trend, that of placing greater reliance on primary health care structures for antimalarial activities. Sometimes this is successful, especially when these are single-purpose interventions delivered through community workers (Mburu et al., 1987; Ruebush et al., 1990); but often insufficient attention is paid to adapting policies to resource constraints and to the competing demands on health staff, who become multipurpose workers. Jeffery (1984) described the problems which arose when malaria chemotherapy was incorporated into community-based primary health care schemes; in particular, too many other activities were added on, and resources did not expand to accommodate the additions. Laing (1984) reviewed the experience with chemoprophylaxis in several African countries, and found that an increasing lack of resources made it impossible to ensure regular drug distribution and supervision of the chemoprophylaxis programmes.

Drug regulations may also cause unexpected distortions in drug use. The policy of the national drug supply company in Togo was to sell a minimum of 20 tablets, at about 6 CFA francs each; this was unaffordable for a large number of potential clients who preferred to pay a higher price per tablet for the possibility of buying only a few (Deming et al., 1989). One anthropologist who has studied drug use in detail concludes that the legal regulation that pharmacists sell drugs only in standardized packs, as in Togo, actually works to their advantage. They sell drugs at retail price to street vendors who break the packs down and sell smaller quantities to the poorer segments of the population; the vendors thus undertake the unprofitable part of the retail trade for them while extending their market (Van der Geest, 1987). Ironically, the closer one gets to poorest income groups, the higher the unit price of antimalarial drugs.

The failure of the health service

Even where the policy framework is appropriate, resource constraints may mean that health services are unable to provide an appropriate level of service. The presence of a thriving 'unofficial' drugs market and extensive self-medication often means that the public health services are either inaccessible (either geographically or financially), or of such low quality that they are not patronized. In developing countries, only about 10–15 % of outpatients are seen by a medically qualified person, and the level of education of lower-level health staff may be very basic. Furthermore, at lower-level health facilities there may be no capacity to perform even the most simple laboratory tests. The rapidly

changing picture as regards chloroquine resistance makes up-to-date prescribing information for prescribers, drug dispensers and the public even more
necessary; yet this information is rarely provided. Guyer and Candy, writing in
1979, documented the poor quality of health services and of treatment for
malaria in Cameroon. Overuse of injections with poorly sterilized equipment
and use of expensive injectibles when cheaper, safer oral drugs would be better
and safer, was common. They pointed out that injectible antimalarials are a
source of iatrogenic disease; and that 'the cooking pot with needles and syringes
boiling over a gas fire ... should be seen as a potential hazard to patients' (Guyer
and Candy, 1979). Written in the pre-HIV days of 1979, these cautions are even
more timely today. Ten years later, however, Ndumbe (1989) reported that
many of the same problems were still present in Cameroon, and 63 % of nurses,
and about 50 % of doctors, would prescribe an injection either alone or in
combination with tablets or suppositories. One reason frequently given for
prescribing a given drug was that it was available! Nurses prescribed more
injections than did doctors, and most reported that it was the patient's choice
rather than their own professional judgment that guided their decision
(Ndumbe, 1989). It is important to bear in mind that nurses provide a very high
proportion of treatments for malaria in Cameroon, as elsewhere in Africa; and
even more worrying is that the nurses in Ndumbe's sample were mainly
employed as *instructors* in nursing schools where they teach their own prescription habits to their students.

Overprescription is a major problem. Prescribers frequently do not know the
prices of drugs; many prescribe a large number of drugs in the expectation that
the patients will think they are 'good doctors'. In many countries there is
overlap of the roles of patient and client, where the prescriber benefits either
directly or indirectly from the sale of drugs, and the prescriber thus has an
interest in prescribing the maximum amount of drugs which the patient/client
can afford. Patients, on the other hand, may expect a long prescription to
validate their 'sick role'; yet they rarely fill a long prescription. If the patient is
unable to decide which of the numerous medications is the one he really needs,
he may ask the person behind the counter at the pharmacy, who is in fact the one
who 'prescribes', usually on the basis of what the patient says he can afford. In
Nigeria, when the cost was between 1 and 9 naira, a prescription was filled in
83 % of cases; but when the cost exceeded 20 naira, only 21 % of prescriptions
were filled (Isenalumhe and Oviawe, 1988). Overprescription can also encourage self-medication. In Pikine, Dakar, the average prescription from a dispensary cost 5200 CFA francs or nearly US$20 (but from a private doctor, as much
as 14 000 CFA francs) but most households received less than 30 000 CFA
francs per month. As a result, most households chose to self-medicate with drugs
bought from market sellers (Fassin, 1986).

Glik and her colleagues found that rural mothers in Guinea who lived far
from health services used health care much less and delayed longer in treating

their children for malaria than did mothers who lived near health clinics. The availability of chloroquine at health centres was strongly associated with use of health services (Glik *et al.*, 1989). In other areas people may be less well informed about how to self-medicate, however; in The Gambia, only 2.3% of mothers would have given chloroquine if they thought their child had malaria but 79% would have given aspirin or paracetamol. This was improved by an education campaign (Menon *et al.*, 1988).

Economic constraints and lack of cash

Governments are increasingly asking their populations to pay for services or for drugs, or for both. If such user charges are well designed and *affordable*, they can have a positive impact on rational use of drugs. However, there is a growing body of evidence to show that often user charges have four types of negative impact that are relevant to malaria control (WHO, 1990):

(1) Utilization of health facilities declines, with the cash-poor segments of the population, especially women and children, accounting for proportionally more of the decline.
(2) Self-medication from 'unofficial' sources increases, since these sources are willing to sell single tablets of drugs at a lower overall cost (although unit costs are higher).
(3) Those patients who continue to frequent health services demand better service; but where there is a flat fee for service unrelated to the consumption of drugs, patients' demand for 'better service' often expresses itself in terms of 'more drugs'. This may lead to pressure on the prescriber for inappropriate quantities or forms (i.e. injections) of drugs. These drugs may then be hoarded for future use or may be sold to others for self-medication.
(4) People cannot find the cash at the times of year when malaria is more prevalent, i.e. during the rainy season just before the harvest.

These problems, and their importance for the malaria control effort, are illustrated by the recent experience of Ashanti-Akim district in Ghana, where a large proportion of outpatient consultations are for malaria (44% at one health centre). Fees increased steeply in June 1985 and the impact was felt immediately. Attendance at health stations dropped to a quarter of 1984 levels, and while the large urban-based stations had recovered two and a half years later, small rural-based stations are still well below half their previous levels of utilization (Waddington and Enyimayew, 1989). But while patient demand had dropped, the quantities of drugs supplied remained the same, resulting in a high wastage of antimalarial drugs. On average, each patient attending the clinic, regardless of age or diagnosis, received up to eight tablets of chloroquine, 29 ml of chloroquine syrup, and 0.5 ml of chloroquine injection (Waddington and Enyimayew, 1989).

Further research on drug use and on the reasons for the decline in attendance at rural health facilities in Ashanti-Akim was undertaken. Many people found the fees too high and instead turned to self-medication at local shops and market sellers, since they could obtain small amounts of drugs there which were cheaper than the fees at the health services. If self-medication failed, patients would go for treatment on about the fourth or fifth day of their illness. Cost considerations caused them to delay their use of government facilities until they were sure the illness was not self-limiting or curable with simple drugs. Ironically, despite the greater incidence of disease, especially malaria, fee collection was at its lowest during the rainy season, because farmers were most likely to be short of cash just before the harvest; and the government fiscal year and budget processes meant that facilities would be most likely to be out of stock of frequently used drugs during the first two quarters of the year (Waddington and Enyimayew, 1989).

The seasonality of malaria means that cash for drug purchases is needed at exactly the time of year when cash is most scarce. Malaria occurs during the rainy season when cash income from the previous harvest is exhausted. Cham *et al.* (1987) found in The Gambia that the rainy season was the time of maximum hunger, work and poverty; cash availability after seven years of drought was so low that many villagers did not have enough cash to purchase chloroquine from the village health workers. If cash was required for health care, the less privileged would either be excluded or would have to beg for cash from their patron or a former master (Cham *et al.*, 1987). Lack of cash was also a problem in rural Malawi, where a drug sales scheme was providing chloroquine at a very low price; but even though there was a malaria epidemic, people could not find the cash to purchase the chloroquine and the drugs eventually had to be given away free or they would have expired (Richardson, 1990).

The 'time cost' of seeking care for malaria is also highest during the rainy season. The workload of the villagers, including village health workers (both men and women) during the rainy season is at its peak; they are often in their fields and therefore not available when the villagers seek them out (Cham *et al.*, 1987). Seasonality hits the poorer groups even harder than the rich; in Kenya, for the poorest 20% of the population, an hour during the rainy season was nearly eight times more valuable than an hour during the dry season (Mwabu, 1988). As a result, for a poor person the cost of seeking care is much higher during the rainy season in terms of both the loss of time which would otherwise be devoted to productive work and in the general low availability of cash needed to pay for transportation, drugs, medical fees, etc.

Consequences of self-medication

Probably the most common, and the most serious, consequence of unsuccessful self-medication is delay in seeking treatment. As noted above, a two-day delay in seeking further treatment following self-medication would not be unusual. In

Thailand people came to the malaria clinics after an average of 7.8 days after onset of symptoms, and most of them had self-medicated before seeking care at the clinics (Somkid, 1983). In Togo only 17% of children with malaria seen in health facilities were seen on the first day of fever (Deming et al., 1989). Unfortunately, with malaria a delay of a few days can prove fatal; in The Gambia the mean duration of symptoms in children who died of malaria was only 2.8 days, and half of the children had been ill for two days or less (Greenwood et al., 1987). In a sample of 1323 paediatric deaths from malaria in Kinshasa, Zaïre, 62% occurred in the emergency ward before admission to hospital (Greenberg et al., 1989). Similarly, in Malawi 28% of a group of 96 children with cerebral malaria had been ill less than 24 hours before presenting to the hospital; and 58% had had antimalarials before arrival at hospital (Taylor and Molyneux, 1988).

There are many possible causes of delay in seeking treatment. The availability of different brands of chloroquine on the market may cause confusion in self-medication and in particular under- or overdosing, and also result in delay in seeking treatment. People might start self-medication with Nivaquine, and when the condition did not improve, they might switch to Resochin — another form of chloroquine marketed by a different company. In the meantime the illness may have progressed. The fact that the tablets are different sizes (100 mg and 150 mg base) and in different packaging might also suggest to the layman that they are different drugs. People are often poorly informed about correct doses; in Zimbabwe the doses people reported for malaria prophylaxis varied from 300 mg base every two months to 300 mg base daily, with only 16% of urban and 31% of rural people consuming the proper dose (Stein et al., 1988).

The wide variety of brands is confusing to health staff as well. In Tanzania a survey found that a main cause of underdosing with chloroquine was confusion over doses, especially with injectible chloroquine. This is not surprising; ten different brands of injectible chloroquine in different strengths (sometimes labelled in terms of the salt, sometimes in terms of the base), from seven different manufacturers in six countries, were in use in the health services. Health staff would just become familiar with one brand when that one would run out and be substituted by another one; this is a common problem, especially when most drugs are donated. Another cause of underdosing was scarcity of drugs, in particular chloroquine tablets (Lyimo, 1987).

The growing extent of chloroquine resistance may also cause a delay in seeking further treatment; parents, and lower-level health staff, may not realize the extent of chloroquine resistance, and that the dose which cured malaria a few years ago is no longer completely reliable. In Kinshasa, Zaïre, there was a striking increase in malaria morbidity and mortality between 1982 and 1986, which may be related to the rapid intensification of chloroquine resistance over that period; in 1982 no cases of resistance had been detected but, by 1986, 82% of *Plasmodium falciparum* parasites isolated from children at Mama Yemo hospital were resistant *in vitro* to chloroquine. Blood samples were collected from 140 malaria patients presenting to the emergency ward, and 92% had evidence of recent intake of chloroquine and/or quinine (Greenberg *et al.*, 1989). Parents and lower-level health workers may have delayed treatment or referral in the expectation that chloroquine would cure the malaria.

Another possible consequence of self-medication is overdose of antimalarial drugs. As noted above, a large proportion of patients seen in hospital have previously self-medicated; and in a survey in Nigeria 50% of children attending an outpatient clinic for malaria had 'therapeutic' levels of chloroquine in their blood (WHO, 1990). Busy hospital staff may fail to take a detailed history and may consequently administer a treatment, i.e. a parenteral loading dose of quinine, that results in a peak at the same time as an earlier dose of chloroquine is reaching its peak — with potentially serious results (WHO, 1990).

Finally, self-medication with antimalarials may be used for conditions that are not malaria at all, and other causes of fever will go undetected or untreated. Health staff working in some parts of Africa report that some patients who complain of 'malaria' and have previously self-medicated are actually suffering · from AIDS-related illnesses which cause fever and body pains.

The disadvantages of self-medication with antimalarials, therefore, are numerous, with the most obvious being delay in seeking further care, the development of resistance and the risks of incorrect dosing. Some authors feel that this is justification for prohibiting the sale of drugs over the counter (Stein *et al.*, 1988), whereas others consider that the benefits may outweigh the risks (Fassin, 1988; Raynal, 1985; Menon *et al.*, 1988). In any case, prohibition is not a realistic option; it is a fact of life in the developing world.

Options for improving the situation

Drugs used for self-medication constitute an important part of the health resources available at local level. It is clear that self-medication is not likely to disappear in the foreseeable future and there are reasons to believe that it is on the increase. What options are available to take advantage of this situation?

Match policy with reality

It is essential to ensure that policies regarding treatment of malaria and use of antimalarial drugs are realistic and feasible within resource constraints, both human and financial. There seems to be growing recognition of the many constraints; the most recent WHO technical report of chemotherapy of malaria is entitled *Practical Chemotherapy of Malaria*; its predecessor was called *Advances in Malaria Chemotherapy* (WHO, 1984). The difference is more than semantic; the first document assumes that antimalarials are used within the context of malarial control programmes, whereas the second assumes no such thing and acknowledges the widespread use of self-medication. The recent document also makes several practical suggestions, such as the need to develop a suppository form of antimalarial for use at lower levels of health services when oral therapy is impossible but where referral is also impossible.

Improve health services

Although major efforts are being made to improve the health services, it is worth noting that poor health services, and in particular insufficient and irregular drug supply, are the major barriers to improvement of the treatment of malaria. While we are 'waiting for the vaccine' it is sobering to note how poorly we have managed with the tools available to date. There is no guarantee that availability of a vaccine would do anything at all to reduce morbidity and mortality from malaria in remote rural areas or among the urban poor.

Restrict drug availability

Attempts to restrict drugs to prescription only have rarely succeeded in developing countries. In the private sector the designation 'prescription only' merely increases the client demand and makes it more difficult to restrict its use, especially in countries that lack the resources actually to inspect pharmacies and drug sellers. In Brazil the inscription 'for sale on doctor's prescription' became more of a quality certificate than a restrictive measure (Haak, 1988). In Sierra Leone the additional difficulty of obtaining a prescription-only medicine enhanced its value (Bledsoe and Goubaud, 1985). The public's awareness of the possibility of chloroquine resistance, which may be enhanced by the private sector advertising and contact with pharmacy employees, may act in favour of the sale of newer antimalarials. In Papua New Guinea, however, there has been some success with restricting the use of certain antimalarials within the health system, to specific levels of health care; sulfadoxine-pyrimethamine is available 'only on prescription' and is authorized only to health subcentre level for treatment of severe and resistant malaria, whereas quinine injection is limited in quantity at lower levels of the health services to prevent overuse (Pyakalyia, 1989).

Investigate the social, economic and cultural dimensions of malaria

To date, research in human behaviour, in particular the use of antimalarial and other drugs, has been relatively rare, so results of such studies have not had a great impact (Litsios, 1989). Yet such research is essential to an understanding of why programmes succeed or fail. Take the example of a chloroquine prophylaxis programme for pregnant women in Malawi that failed. Sociological investigation revealed that the bitter taste of chloroquine was associated with traditional herbs which cause abortion, and pregnant women were advised to avoid all bitter medicine during pregnancy. Provision of coated tablets significantly increased compliance (Heymann *et al.*, 1990). Similarly, Glik *et al.* (1989) found in Guinea that use of maternal chemoprophylaxis was affected by the local knowledge that a large dose of chloroquine would produce an abortion, which created a perception that the drug was dangerous for pregnant women. In addition, an understanding of human behaviour as it relates to malaria and using up-to-date and culturally acceptable means of communication, are essential if the use of antimalarials is to be improved and if measures to inform and educate the general public are to be effective.

Keep malaria treatments affordable for the target population

Treatment of malaria has a strong 'public good' aspect, and free treatment could be justified on the same economic grounds as provision of immunizations or maternal and child care. However, the economic situation of many endemic countries makes it unlikely that malaria treatment can be provided free, especially given the costs of drugs and the large numbers of cases to be treated. If therefore there is to be a charge for antimalarial treatment, the price should be nominal. Even nominal fees may be unaffordable during a malaria epidemic, so provision for free treatment must be made.

Recent trends in the pricing of antimalarials indicate that despite the development of several promising new drugs for the most part their prices (e.g. US$5 per treatment for halofrantrine, US$5 for mefloquine unless purchased through WHO) put them beyond the reach of many people in endemic countries, particularly in Africa, where *annual* per capita drug expenditures rarely exceed US$5. The prices of new antimalarials should be kept as low as possible, and in any case below US$1 per treatment episode, if they are to be available where needed. The implicit use of price as a rationing measure and for determination of level of use should be examined. Research into ways of preserving chloroquine as a first-line drug, including reversal of chloroquine resistance using low-cost adjuvant drugs, could prove very useful.

There is a dual market for any new antimalarial drug or therapy, including a vaccine; one part of the market includes about 20 million affluent travellers, including military personnel, diplomats, tourists, businessmen, and the wealthy elite of developing countries, who can afford to pay a high price for antimalarials. The other market, the 2000 million poor people living in endemic countries, have a very limited ability to pay. If past experience with antimalarial drugs is any guide, there will be a major difficulty in making any new vaccine available at a price they can afford. It is not clear, therefore, that availability of a vaccine in itself will have any impact *at all* on morbidity and mortality from malaria.

More rational patterns of self-medication and unofficial use could be encouraged

Families could be encouraged to keep a small stock of chloroquine for full radical treatment (Menon *et al.*, 1988); this would need to be accompanied by instructions on dosage, as well as clear, unambiguous guidance on when to seek further treatment, bearing in mind that the referral facility may be a day or more away. Schoolchildren (often more literate than their parents) could be used to disseminate information about antimalarials and their use. Rural storekeepers, market sellers, and other 'unofficial' drug distributors could be provided with simple information on use of antimalarials; in the past they have proved receptive to such information and recognition. If their activities in distribution of antimalarials could be improved, the network for distribution would be extended to a much lower level than is possible working through official control programmes or government health facilities. Unfortunately, the fact that the activities of 'unofficial' drug sellers are illegal makes it difficult to work with them to improve their knowledge of correct usage and dosage (Deming *et al.*, 1989; Fassin, 1988). Illiterate volunteers with only two days' training have been used for malaria case detection and treatment with success in Guatemala (Ruebush *et al.*, 1990) and in Kenya (Mburu *et al.*, 1987).

Keeping knowledge up to date

Prescribers and the public at large need to be kept up to date on treatment of malaria, and in particular on the local situation with regard to chloroquine resistance. At present much of their information comes from representatives of pharmaceutical companies who may tend to exaggerate the need for new antimalarials. The essential drugs programmes in operation in many countries could be used to distribute not only drugs but information as well, with malaria guidelines being included in prescribers' manuals, and in drug ration kits, and discussed at prescriber training seminars. Less conventional methods could be used to reach the public, including radio and television, print media, literacy classes, advertising, and so on.

Conclusion

It is hoped that the reader is now convinced that the distribution and use of antimalarial drugs does not follow a clear, tidy logic, as is sometimes assumed, and that indeed it is 'not a pretty picture' if one is looking for clarity and logic. However, it is a fascinating illustration of the complexity of human behaviour and the interaction between medical science and culture. An appreciation and understanding of this complexity will increase the possibility of finding lasting solutions to some of the problems raised. While we are 'waiting for the vaccine', it is worth pondering how we will solve some of these same problems which, inevitably, will arise when a malaria vaccine becomes a reality.

References

Note: this chapter draws on an earlier paper (MAP/SGCM/WP89.4) prepared by the author for the WHO Scientific Group on the Chemotherapy of Malaria, June 1989, the report of which was recently published as Practical Chemotherapy of Malaria, *Technical Report Series* 805, World Health Organization, Geneva, 1990.

Bledsoe CH and Goubaud MF (1985) The reinterpretation of Western pharmaceuticals among the Mende of Sierra Leone. *Social Science and Medicine, 21*, 275–282

Cham K, MacCormack C, Touray A and Bai-Deh S (1987) Social organization and political factionalism: PHC in The Gambia. *Health Policy and Planning, 2*, 214–226

Deming M, Gayibor A, Murphy K, Jones TS and Karsa T (1989) The home treatment of febrile children with anti-malarial drugs in Togo. *Bulletin of the World Health Organization, 67*, 695–700

Fassin D (1986) La vente illicite des médicaments au Sénégal. *Politique Africaine, 23*, 123–130

Fassin D (1988) Illicit sale of pharmaceuticals in Africa: sellers and clients in the suburbs of Dakar. *Tropical and Geographical Medicine, 40*, 166–170

Glik DC, Ward WB, Gordon A and Haba F (1989) Malaria treatment practices among mothers in Guinea. *Journal of Health and Social Behaviour, 30*, 421–435

Gomes M and Salazar NP (1990) Chemotherapy: principles in practice—a case study of the Philippines. *Social Science and Medicine, 30*, 789–796

Greenberg AE, Ntumbanzondo M, Ntula N, Mawa L, Howell J and Davachi F (1989) Hospital-based surveillance of malaria-related pediatric morbidity and mortality in Kinshasa, Zaire. *Bulletin of the World Health Organization, 67*, 189–196

Greenwood BM, Bradley AK, Greenwood AM, Byass P, Jammeh K, Marsh K, Tulloch S, Oldfield FSJ and Hayes R (1987) Mortality and morbidity from malaria among children in a rural area of the Gambia, West Africa. *Transactions of the Royal Society of Tropical Medicine and Hygiene, 81*, 478–486

Guyer B and Candy D (1979) Injectable anti-malarial therapy in tropical Africa: iatrogenic disease and wasted medical resources. *Transactions of the Royal Society of Tropical Medicine and Hygiene, 73*, 230–232

Haak H (1988) Pharmaceuticals in two Brazilian villages: lay practices and perceptions. *Social Science and Medicine, 27*, 1415–1427

Heymann DL, Steketee RW, Wirima JJ, McFarland DA, Khoromana CO and Campbell CC (1990) Antenatal chloroquine chemoprophylaxis in Malawi: chloroquine resistance, compliance, protective efficacy, and cost. *Transactions of the Royal Society of Tropical Medicine and Hygiene, 84*, 496–498

Isenalumhe AE and Oviawe O (1988) Polypharmacy: its cost burden and barrier to medical care in a drug-oriented health care system. *International Journal of Health Services, 18*, 335–342

Jeffery GM (1984) The role of chemotherapy in malaria control through primary health care: constraints and future prospects. *Bulletin of the World Health Organization, 62*, 49–53

Laing, AG (1984) The impact of malaria chemoprophylaxis in Africa with special reference to Madagascar, Cameroon, and Senegal. *Bulletin of the World Health Organization, 62*, 41–48

Litsios S (1989) *Public Information and Education in Malaria Control: Need for Research and Development*, 22nd meeting of the Steering Committee of the Scientific Working Group on Applied Field Research in Malaria, WHO/FDR, April (unpublished)

Lyimo, EO (1987) Chloroquine administration in the treatment of malaria with reference to brands, specifications, and dosage: a survey in Northeast Tanzania. *East African Medical Journal, 64,* 551–557

MacCormack CP and Lwihula G (1983) Failure to participate in a malaria chemosuppression programme: North Mara, Tanzania. *Journal of Tropical Medicine and Hygiene, 86,* 99–107

Mburu FM, Spencer HC and Kaseje DCO (1987) Changes in sources of treatment occurring after inception of a community-based malaria control programme in Saradidi, Kenya. *Annals of Tropical Medicine and Parasitology, 81,* 105–110

Menon A, Joof D, Rowan KM and Greenwood BM (1988) Maternal administration of chloroquine: an unexplored aspect of malaria control. *Journal of Tropical Medicine and Hygiene, 91,* 49–54

Mills AJ (1990) The economic evaluation of malaria control technologies: the case of Nepal. Paper presented to the Second World Conference of Health Economics, Zurich, 10–14 September 1990

Mwabu G (1988) Seasonality and the shadow price of time, and the effectiveness of tropical disease control programmes. In Herrin AN and Rosenfield PL (eds) *Economics, Health and Tropical Diseases*, University of the Philippines School of Economics, Manila

Ndumbe PM (1989) Curative and preventive treatment of uncomplicated malaria in public health institutions in Cameroon. *European Journal of Epidemiology, 5,* 183–188

Pyakalyia T (1989) Progress and problems in the diagnosis and treatment of malaria and development of an effective referral system in Papua New Guinea. *Papua New Guinea Medical Journal, 32,* 167–170

Raynal AL (1985) Use of over-the-counter medications in rural Matabeleland, Zimbabwe: the case for upgrading the dispensing skills of rural storekeepers. *Central African Journal of Medicine, 31,* 92–97

Richardson S (1990) *Charging for Malaria Treatment in Rural Malawi: Recovering Costs or Restricting a Control Strategy?* Unpublished MSc dissertation, London School of Hygiene and Tropical Medicine

Ruebush TK, Zeissig R, Godoy HA and Klein HE (1990) Use of illiterate volunteer workers for malaria case detection and treatment. *Annals of Tropical Medicine and Parasitology, 84,* 119–125

Somkid Kaewsonthi (1983) *Cost and performance appraisal of malaria surveillance and monitoring measures: final report*, WHO/TDR, May

Stein CM, Gora NP and Macheka BM (1988) Self-medication with chloroquine for malaria prophylaxis in urban and rural Zimbabweans. *Tropical and Geographical Medicine, 40,* 264–268

Taylor TE and Molyneux ME (1988) Cerebral malaria in children: presenting features and prognosis. *Malawi Medical Quarterly, 5,* 3–11

Van der Geest S (1987) Self-care and the informal sale of drugs in South Cameroon. *Social Science and Medicine, 25,* 293–305

Waddington C and Enyimayew KA (1989) A price to pay: the impact of user charges in Ashanti-Akim district, Ghana. *International Journal of Health Planning and Management, 4,* 17

World Health Organization (1984) Advances in malaria chemotherapy: report of a WHO scientific group. *Technical Report Series* 711, Geneva

World Health Organization (1988) *The World Drug Situation.* Geneva

World Health Organization (1990) Practical chemotherapy of malaria: report of a WHO scientific group. *Technical Report Series* 805, Geneva

WORKSHOP REPORT AND RECOMMENDATIONS
RAPPORTEUR: ALBERTO ALZATE

Health authorities have an increasing role in defining national policies for distribution and use of antimalarial drugs. There is also a need for lists of essential (available?) drugs in all countries; the support of national governments and of international agencies in achieving these objectives is required during the coming decade.

International purchasing mechanisms should be created to relieve countries of the pressures of fluctuations in the rate of exchange and the availability of foreign currency, and to stimulate the pharmaceutical industry to supply the drugs required.

Improvements in existing capacity for diagnosis and treatment are required; hence resources, including drugs, should be targeted on high-risk groups.

The strengthening of regulatory mechanisms directed towards quality control of medicines, prices and improvement in knowledge about prescription among health personnel are very important not only in the public sector but also in the growing sector of private pre-paid medicine prevalent in some countries.

The educational policies designed to provide information and training for mothers, health professionals, drug sellers and traditional healers should be oriented towards use of early and appropriate measures for therapy, including treatment in the home.

The establishment of mechanisms for monitoring and surveillance of the whole process of drug supply and use is vitally necessary. These should include household surveys, and economic, social and epidemiological evaluations.

Several neglected areas of research should be supported. These include behavioural aspects of self-diagnosis, home treatment, choices available for health care, natural drugs, and the role of traditional healers in diagnosis of malaria.

The economics of malaria control

Anne Mills

London School of Hygiene and Tropical Medicine, and London School of Economics, UK

Introduction

Economics is 'the study of how people and society end up choosing, with or without the use of money, to employ scarce productive resources that could have alternative uses, to produce various commodities and distribute them for consumption, now or in the future, among various persons or groups in society. It analyses the costs and benefits of improving patterns of resource allocation' (Samuelson, 1976). Economics can thus be seen as the study of scarcity and choice, and is relevant wherever resource scarcity or scope for choice exists — such as health (Lee and Mills, 1985).

While — perhaps in the interests of respectability — health economists may like to trace their discipline back several centuries (Klarman, 1979; Rosenthal, 1979), most health economics theories, concepts and techniques have been developed in the past two decades. It is not surprising therefore that the literature on any one topic — such as malaria control — is limited. Moreover, in the health economics literature concerned with developing countries, the heavy involvement of donor agencies has meant an emphasis on certain areas of health economics. In relation to malaria control, this has led to an extremely selective literature, focusing on the benefits of malaria control (or the 'costs' of malaria), and (to a lesser extent) on the costs and cost-effectiveness of malaria control activities.

This chapter describes what is known about the economics of malaria control, identifying what is not known and ought to be investigated and considering the major issues that arise, and concludes with some comments on the economic choices that would be presented by a malaria vaccine, were one to become available.

The economics of malaria control

The economics of malaria control is much broader than simply the application of techniques of cost-effectiveness and cost-benefit analysis, and is concentrated on five areas of concern:

(1) Who gets malaria?
(2) What are the resource costs of malaria?
(3) What determines an individual's or a community's demand for malaria control measures and treatment?
(4) What are the characteristics of the various means to satisfy this demand, i.e. of the supply of control and treatment measures?
(5) What policies follow from the comparison of the costs and consequences of different means of supply?

These are considered in turn below.

The determinants of malaria transmission

Studies are at present too few to produce general conclusions, particularly since findings from one location may not be relevant to another. Moreover, many conceptual and methodological difficulties, of formulating a model of determinants and testing it, remain to be resolved (Birdsall, 1990; Behrman and Deolikar, 1988). This is none-the-less an important research area since better information will allow more efficient targeting of limited resources on high-risk groups.

Presently available results are unsurprising. Occupation and worksite, and to a lesser extent socioeconomic characteristics, are shown to be risk factors in several studies from Latin America (Fernandez and Sawyer, 1988; Castro and Mokate, 1988; Banguero, 1984). In Thailand, younger people, migrant workers and those whose work takes them into the forest were found to be particularly at risk (Fungladda et al., 1987). Vosti (1990) did not find the wide interpersonal differences in malaria prevalence and association with socioeconomic and environmental factors found by Fernandez and Sawyer: simply living and working in a high-risk area was the most powerful determinant of the risk of infection. Since Vosti's sample was of miners only, at their worksites, this finding is unsurprising.

These studies have so far shed little light on whether and how individuals adapt their behaviour to influence their risk. Researchers have included direct or indirect measures of people's knowledge of malaria in equations describing the risk of infection, in the hope that if they prove significant (and appropriately signed) health education would offer promise of influencing individuals to adopt preventive measures. Only the study by Vosti (1990) produced suggestive results, finding weak but negative relationships between reported malaria prevalence and age, information about and/or experience with malaria prior to arriving at the goldmine site, and miners' origins and previous occupations, which he interpreted as suggesting scope for individuals to reduce their risk.

The resource costs of malaria

The resource costs of malaria are of two main types. First there are the costs to the health system of coping with the disease—the costs of treatment and prevention (often termed direct costs). Secondly there are costs that can be expressed in terms of production (often termed indirect costs). These can be short term or long term. Short-term production consequences follow from reduction in labour supply due to morbidity and mortality and in the productivity of labour, and constraints on the supply of land. Long-term production consequences include demographic effects on per capita consumption, labour supply and capital formation; unwillingness to take risks and innovate; and reduced intellectual development of children. It cannot be emphasized too strongly that these resource costs do not reflect the value of ill health per se (though many of the studies do not make this clear) since they describe only its more material consequences.

The great majority of studies on the resource costs of malaria concentrate on treatment costs and days of work lost, leaving aside the more intractable issues of demographic consequences, attitudes to risk and innovation and effect on intellectual development. Table 1 summarizes the methods and findings of these studies (those marked with an asterisk compare savings in resource costs with the cost of control to estimate a cost-benefit ratio—see later).

Treatment costs are typically estimated on the basis of very weak data on public sector costs, still weaker figures on private expenditure and speculative assumptions of the proportion of cases who seek treatment. There is a tendency to assume a seemingly exaggerated figure for this proportion, and then multiply it by presumed incidence and cost per treatment to obtain an enormous figure for the total direct costs of malaria.

A similar tendency to exaggerate can be deduced in Table 1 from the enormous variation in days of disability per malaria episode assumed (or measured) in the various studies. Since days of disability lost will depend on such factors as the parasite species, immune status of the population, frequency of attacks per individual and whether or not the episode is treated, comparison between the studies must be undertaken cautiously. However, it is notable that those studies which measure days of disability from their own surveys (e.g. Conly, 1975; Mason and Hobbs, 1977; Miller, 1958; Mills, 1989; Picard and Mills, 1990) tend to find lower values than the other studies which rely on assumptions, suggesting a tendency for the latter to be exaggerated.

Most studies ignore the chain of events that will determine whether or not a period of illness will lead to a loss of production. The main links in the chain are as follows.

Infection to disability and debility

Not all those infected may be disabled or debilitated (especially where adults have a considerable degree of immunity): for example, Brohult et al. (1981)

Table 1 Measurement and valuation of direct (treatment costs saved) and indirect (production gains) benefits from malaria control[a]

Reference	Group/ area studied	Valuation of treatment costs	Disability and debility (days/episode)	Method of valuation of days lost
Barlow (1968)*	Sri Lanka	Reduction in public and private treatment costs assumed to increase saving and investment: values used not stated	Not stated: based on malariologists' opinions and data from household survey of morbidity	Based on estimated elasticity of output with respect to skilled and unskilled labour
Bhombore et al. (1952)	2 villages in India	Expenditure/family/year on malaria compared pre- and post-spraying in sprayed and control villages	Not reported in study	Wage rate for hired labour
Bruce-Chwatt (1963)	Psychiatric patients, Lagos	Not valued	2.6 days (untreated) 1 attack/person/2 years	Not valued
Castro and Mokate (1988)	Cunday, Colombia	Not valued	Analysed by occupational group and year; e.g. labourers 7–11 days (from survey)	Hourly wage
Chernin (1954)	Jute mill, India	Not valued	Average of 2.1 days (from survey)	Not valued
Cohn (1973)	India	Not valued due to lack of data but considered to be sizeable	Discussed but not quantified	Discussed but not valued
Conly (1975)	Area of Paraguay	Not discussed	5.4 days (from survey)	Not valued directly
Gazin et al. (1988)	Factory in Burkina Faso	Not valued	3.5 days (from survey)	Not valued
Ghana Health Assessment Project Team (1981)	Ghana	Not valued	7 days	Not valued
Hall and Wilks (1967)	Tanzania	Not valued	1.16 days/person/year	Not valued
Kaewsonthi (1988)	2 zones in Thailand	Reported travel, time and treatment costs	5.3 and 5.5 days	Minimum wage and actual average daily income

Khan (1966)*	W. Pakistan	Estimated private expenditure per case	10 days (disability) plus 10 (debility)	'Average product of labour'
Kuhner (1971)	Thailand	Not valued	15 days	Marginal product of labour year from Cobb–Douglas production function
Livadas and Athanassatos (1963)	Greece	Cost of antimalarials, private medical care of 1/6 of cases and hospitalization of 1/60 of cases	6 days	Daily wage
Mason and Hobbs (1977)	Area of El Salvador	Not valued	2.9 days (*P. falciparum*); 2.4 days (*P. vivax*) (survey)	Not valued
Miller (1958)	20 W. African men	Not valued	4.2 days/episode; 6.5 days/year; 3 workdays lost/year	Not valued
Mills (1989)	Nepal: 3253 cases in 6 districts 867 case-control pairs in 2 areas	Reported payment plus assumptions on how would change without control	9.4 days/worker (range by district 6.1–14.5) (survey) 3.8 district 1; 9.3 district 2 (from survey); plus further days partly disabled	Reported financial losses due to malaria episode
Niazi (1969)*	Iraq	Cost of drugs for all cases; of hospital care for 3 days for 10%	7 days	Daily wage
Nur and Mahran (1988)	Gezira, Sudan	Reported payment	6 (disability, from survey) plus 5 days at 50% productivity	Not valued
Ortiz (1968)*	Paraguay	Not assessed	44 days	Assumed value of output per man day by agricultural sector
Picard and Mills (1990)	Nepal	See Mills (1989)	Extra 5.3 days compared to control, plus further effect after perceived recovery	Not valued
Quo (1959)	Philippines	Not known	7 days	Minimum weekly wage
Ramaiah (1980)	India	Total cases × unit cost of outpatient, hospital and private care	5 days/person/year	Income per capita adjusted for sex differences and employment rates
Rao and Bhombore (1956)	Mysore state, India	Not assessed	6 days	Daily wage

continued overleaf

Table 1 (*continued*)

Reference	Group/ area studied	Valuation of treatment costs	Disability and debility (days/episode)	Method of valuation of days lost
Ruberu (1977)	Sri Lanka	90% of cases × outpatient cost; 10% of cases × hospital cost for 3 days	5 days	Average earning capacity of self-employed rural farm hand
Russell and Menon (1942)	2 Indian villages	Reported payment for treatment and religious ceremonies	Per person over 21: 9.7 days (village 1), 20.7 days (village 2) (from survey)	Reported earnings losses
San Pedro (1967-8)*	Philippines	Estimated cost of outpatient care (doctor, lab tests, drugs) × number of cases	7 days (disability) plus 20% loss in working efficiency for 6 weeks	Legal minimum wage for agricultural workers
Shepard et al. (1990)	Africa	Unit cost × data and assumptions on % treated	3.5–6 days for severe malaria; 1.7–3.5 for carer	Various methods, e.g. value of output, average income per capita
Sinton (1935/6)	India	Discussed. Average cost per case × no. of cases	7 days (disability) plus 10% loss in working efficiency over 1 year	Average monthly wage rate weighted for different earnings by sex
Van Dine (1916)	Louisiana, USA	Not assessed	6.42 equivalent adult days per case plus 25% loss of working efficiency in crop season	Days of work actually required but not available valued in terms of loss of cotton
Vosti (1990)	Goldminers at 4 sites in Brazil	Reported payment	mean 9.8 days; median 5.9 (from survey)	Wage paid to replacement worker
Wright (1977)	Indonesia	67% of cases × chloroquine cost; 33% × clinic cost; 6% × hospital cost for 5 days	6 days	Employed (61%) × daily wage; underemployed (30%) × .5 of wage; unemployed (9%) not valued

* These studies estimate a cost–benefit ratio.
[a] Those studies which estimate the 'burden of disease' treat these as 'costs'; those which assess the value of control treat them as 'benefits' (averted costs).

found no difference in work capacity between Liberian men in holo- and meso-endemic areas and between infected and uninfected men; Pehrson *et al.* (1984) found no difference in the work capacity of industrial workers who received malaria prophylaxis and those who did not. On the other hand, not all those who lose work time will have been infected (for example, carers).

Disability and debility to days of production lost

Not all those disabled would have been productively employed in market or non-market production, especially at slack times of the year. Moreover, recent studies have shown that production loss may be reduced by substitute workers from within the household or outside it, though it is unclear to what extent the substitute workers in consequence reduce leisure time or less urgent or valuable production tasks. Bonilla de Castro (1985) found in an area of Colombia that the work of ill members was virtually always taken over by non-salaried family members, who continued at the same time their normal activities. Mills (1989) also found in Nepal that the great majority of the study households coped with the malaria episode without difficulty by drawing on household reserves of labour, primarily of adults rather than children, and over 70% of households did not think household production would suffer as a result of the malaria episode. On the other hand, the same data set suggested malaria may continue to reduce work time even after the patient feels completely recovered (Picard and Mills, 1990), though it was impossible to check whether the patient worked harder after recovery in compensation. Amongst Gezira tenants in the Sudan, 62% of the loss of work hours due to malaria was compensated for by family members, primarily women and children, though at the expense of household activities and schooling (Nur and Mahran, 1988).

Days of production lost to the value of production lost

Calculation of production lost and its value should allow for the low marginal value of labour at certain times of the year and the variation in productivity by age and sex, and should include the value of both market and non-market activities. The valuation of non-market activities is difficult (Goldschmidt-Clermont, 1987), and few studies attempt accurate estimates. Many of the studies in Table 1 use some estimate of the average wage, adjusted or unadjusted, thus implicitly assuming the labour market is perfect and that wages reflect marginal product. Others use average product values which, in the presence of declining returns, will be above the marginal value. (The only substantially different approach was that of Kuhner, 1971, who based his estimate on a production function.) Most of these studies value years of life lost due to mortality in a similar fashion, basing the estimate on the average or minimum wage, or annual income per capita. The main exception is Quo (1959), who used the value placed on death by the Philippines Civil Code.

Clearly attempts to quantify production losses due to malaria on the basis of the number of episodes are fraught with difficulty. An alternative approach is to consider production directly. Few studies have attempted this. Conly (1975) found that those families who experienced much malaria gave greater priority to cash crops and slowed down land clearing as compared to families who experienced little malaria. Audibert (1986) found no effect of malaria on the production of rice-growers in Cameroon.

Barlow (1967) took a third approach, which required the assumptions necessary on work-time loss and treatment costs but combined them together with other assumptions in a macro-economic model of the Sri Lankan economy, to evaluate the long-term effect of malaria control on income per capita. The essence of his conclusion is that malaria control encouraged population growth which in the long term led to lower per capita income than would have occurred without malaria control. However, there is considerable controversy over the values of many of the variables in the model.

A review of the evidence that malaria has prevented the cultivation of land, or that malaria control has permitted the exploitation of previously unused land, has highlighted even weaker evidence (Andreano and Helminiak, 1988). For example, claims have been made that malaria control (plus the reduction of other diseases) was the main reason for the settlement and subsequent productivity of the Nepalese Terai; however, for some centuries the Terai, despite malaria, had provided substantial revenue for the ruling classes from the export of forest products and grain (Mills, forthcoming).

Demand for malaria treatment and prevention

The traditional economic model of demand explains the demand for particular goods or services in terms of variables such as price, income, tastes and the prices of other goods and services. Despite strong evidence that individuals do make choices (for example, in their use of private health facilities for malaria treatment despite the existence of 'free' government services, and in their purchase of bednets) little empirical work has been done on the factors influencing demand (for an anthropological study on bednets see MacCormack et al., 1989). Results would be extremely useful to decision makers: for example, an estimate of the price elasticity of demand for bednets could be used to calculate the public cost of the subsidy necessary to achieve a given level of coverage.

Studies of factors influencing demand would also help in ensuring diagnostic and treatment facilities are accessible to those who need them. For example, Ettling et al. (1989) found that women and children were under-represented in malaria clinics, suggesting that the clinics were not serving their needs well, though why is unclear.

Supply of malaria control

There has been virtually no investigation of the characteristics of the supply of malaria control or of alternative technologies, except as part of economic evaluation studies. The emphasis on total costs that this focus encourages has meant neglect of such issues as the mix of inputs, the scope for input substitution, remuneration methods and incentives and the existing and potential role of the private sector. A further shortcoming of existing cost studies is that they estimate costs at a particular level of output. Economic theory suggests that unit costs are unlikely to be constant whatever the output level: there may be increasing or decreasing returns to scale. Thus it is dangerous to extrapolate from a figure which merely represents one point on a cost curve.

Amongst the few studies on the supply of malaria control, Guyer and Candy (1979) have documented waste in health centre prescribing practices, Ruebush *et al.* (1985) the scope for using volunteers to detect malaria, and Rajagopalan and Panicker (1985) the use of environmental management to both control vector breeding and generate income for the community.

Until very recently, it has been assumed that malaria control and treatment should be both financed and provided by the public sector. In the light of severe resource constraints and the current interest in privatization, it is important that arguments be marshalled for and against private-sector involvement. This issue is of particular interest for malaria control since it is, to some extent, a public good, leading to difficulties in the absence of public finance in coordinating individuals to spend an optimal amount. However, public finance does not necessarily imply public provision.

Economic evaluation

The most common forms of economic evaluation (listed in Figure 1) are often confused. Of the four, cost–utility analysis has yet to be used for malaria. Cost analysis simply sums the cost of running a programme, sometimes also including indirect costs (the value of production losses). Cost-effectiveness analysis in its simplest form (that which virtually all developing country studies follow) divides total costs by total health effects (or some proxy indicator of these). Frequently in developed country studies, savings in treatment costs and production which result from health programmes are subtracted from programme costs to produce a 'net cost'. This methodological refinement has tended to blur the distinction between cost-effectiveness analysis and cost–benefit analysis, when benefits in the latter are based on the human capital approach. However, the essential difference is that in cost-effectiveness analysis health effects are retained in natural units whereas in cost–benefit analysis they are converted into monetary terms, whether using the human capital method or another.

Cost–benefit analysis of malaria control

Table 2 gives cost–benefit ratios from malaria control programmes. All use the human capital approach to value benefits and thus focus on the production gains to be obtained by malaria control. Since the cost–benefit ratios are all greater than one, these studies would provide reassuring evidence of the value of malaria control except that they all incorporate assumptions on the direct and indirect cost of malaria, and thus are vulnerable to the criticisms made earlier.

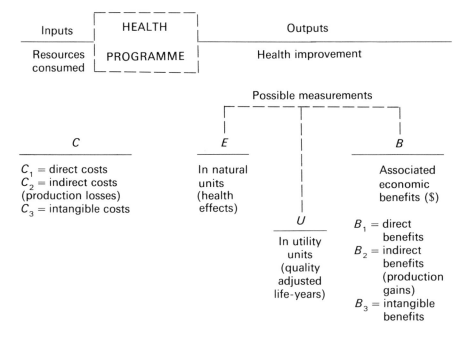

Figure 1   Components of economic evaluation (Source: Drummond and Mills, 1987)

Table 2 Cost–benefit ratios of malaria control programmes

Reference	Country	Method	Cost–benefit ratio
Barlow (1968)	Sri Lanka	Insecticide	146
Griffith *et al.* (1971)	Thailand	Chemoprophylaxis	6.5
Khan (1966)	Pakistan	Eradication programme	4.9
Livandas and Athanassatos (1963)	Greece	Eradication programme	17.3
Niazi (1969)	Iraq	Eradication programme	6.0
Ortiz (1968)	Paraguay	Insecticides	3.6
Ramaiah (1980)	India	Control programme	9.3
San Pedro (1967/8)	Philippines	Eradication programme	2.4
Sudan (1975)	Sudan	Control programme	4.6

Source: Barlow and Grobar (1985); references in table.

Moreover, they also had to make a further set of assumptions on the consequences of prevention. For example, the value of a day's labour may change if a health programme results in a considerable increase in labour days because of declining marginal productivity when one factor of production (labour) is increased but others are not; if people are healthier, they may decide to enjoy more leisure time so production does not increase. If the cost–benefit analysis is done prior to control being started, then assumptions have to be made on the extent of the reduction in malaria and in direct and indirect costs to be expected; if it is done to justify an existing programme, then assumptions have to be made on the amount of malaria and size of costs that would have existed without the programme.

The description of the literature here and earlier must inevitably question whether attempts to assess the costs of malaria and the benefits of malaria control in terms of production gains are worthwhile. Available methods do not match the complexity of the processes by which malaria affects the well-being of households. Moreover, where malaria transmission is most intense, immunity must considerably mitigate the impact of malaria on adult production, and its impact on children is poorly accounted for in the human capital approach (though the impact of child illness on adult production has yet to be fully explored). This view runs counter to that of Birdsall (1990), who argues that

> better documentation of any effects of health status on productivity and income gains could, obviously, increase the interests of policy-makers concerned with economic growth, in health. Ideally it should be possible to compare the benefits of investments in health (as a first step at least in terms of private income gains) to the costs of the investments that generated the additional income gains; such cost-benefit analysis would permit comparison of the rates of return to investments in health with rates of return to alternative investments.

In relation to malaria control at least, such an agenda is highly ambitious.

Cost analysis and cost-effectiveness analysis of malaria control programmes

Cost-effectiveness analysis can be used in two ways. It can produce a cost per health effect (e.g. case prevented) for the entire programme which can then be compared with similar ratios from other health programmes to help decide which are worthwhile (Jamison and Mosley, 1990). The main disadvantages of this approach are that there is as yet no satisfactory common measure of health effects (the strongest contender is 'discounted days of healthy life gained') and little attention is paid to the efficient mix of strategies within the programme. This review focuses on the second way in which cost-effectiveness analysis can be used, namely to compare alternative control methods (Phillips *et al.*, 1990).

Figure 2 provides a framework for reviewing the subjects analysed by malaria control and treatment studies, and indicates the range of strategies that might be assessed. Table 3 briefly describes, in alphabetical order by author, those studies reporting a cost-effectiveness ratio. A very liberal interpretation of cost-effectiveness analysis is applied in order to review a reasonable range of studies. Table 4 summarizes the results of these studies in terms of annual cost per person protected, cost per case prevented and cost per death prevented. Conclusions from this table should be made cautiously since the methods of many of the studies have severe shortcomings: costs are often incomplete and shadow pricing is not employed; very few studies have included time and financial costs of patients and their relatives as well as costs to the government; estimates of effectiveness are often extremely weak except where studies were based on epidemiological trials. Moreover, the studies vary enormously in terms of the circumstances of the study (small-scale trials (e.g. Gandahusada *et al.*, 1984) or national malaria control programmes (e.g. Kaewsonthi, 1988)); and the state of control at the time of the study (a first attempt at control (e.g. Molineaux and Gramiccia, 1980), or a long-established control programme (e.g. Kaewsonthi, 1988) or the entire life of a control programme (e.g. Cohn, 1973 for India, and Barlow, 1968 for Sri Lanka)).

Choice of:

Strategy	Sector	Intervention/technique	Delivery strategy	Target group	Place of intervention	Time of intervention
Prevention Aimed at individual		Impregnated v. unimpregnated bednets	Comparison of case detection and treatment approaches	Case detection and treatment v. mass drug administration to selected groups	Case detection and treatment at home, clinic, volunteer's home, hospital	
Aimed at environment	Design and management of water resource projects; Use of fish	Comparison of insecticides; Comparison of insecticides and environmental management	Comparison of insecticide dosages and coverage	Focal v. full spraying		Number and timing of spray-rounds of insecticide
Diagnosis and treatment		Oral v. injectable drugs; alternative drugs	Diagnosis through malaria clinic or central laboratory; Treatment with or without microscopy; Various means of delivering treatment, e.g. use of PHC network		Treatment at home, clinic or hospital	Prophylaxis v. treatment; Presumptive and radical treatment v. radical treatment alone

Figure 2 Framework for reviewing studies on the cost-effectiveness of malaria control and treatment strategies

Table 3 Description of studies of malaria control reporting a cost-effectiveness ratio

Reference	Group or area studied	Purpose of study	Control methods involved
Barlow (1968)	Sri Lanka: actual data 1947–66; projected data 1976–77	Assess economic impact of malaria eradication	Insecticides; case detection and treatment; surveillance
Bruce-Chwatt and Archibald (1959)	Western Sokoto, Nigeria, 130 000 people	Compare comparative value of 3 insecticides	DDT, BHC, dieldrin; alternative dosages and spray cycles
Bruce-Chwatt (1987)	Non-specific	Assess cost of chemotherapy	Chemotherapy
Cohn (1973)	India, 1950–71	Review costs and benefits of malaria control programme	Insecticides; case detection and treatment; surveillance
El Gaddal et al. (1985)	Gezira, Sudan	Describe costs and effects of spraying	Insecticides
Gandahusada et al. (1984)	3 areas, each c. 50 000 pop., in Central Java, Indonesia, 1980–2	Evaluate full and selective coverage of residual fenitrothion	Insecticides: alternative dosages and coverage
Griffith (1961)	Greece, 1958, national programme	Assess cost of malaria eradication	Surveillance
	Thailand, 1960, field trials	Assess cost of malaria eradication	Surveillance; spraying
	Indonesia, 1961, national programme	Assess cost of malaria eradication	Spraying; spraying and surveillance
	Ceylon, 1960, national programme	Assess cost of malaria eradication	Spraying and surveillance
	Taiwan, 1956 and 1960, national programme	Assess cost of malaria eradication	Spraying; spraying and surveillance; surveillance
	India, 1961, national programme	Assess cost of malaria eradication	Spraying; spraying and surveillance;

Reference	Setting	Objective	Intervention
Hedman et al. (1979)	Mining town in Liberia, pop. 16 000, 1976/7	Evaluate programme	DDT spraying; larvicide measures; chemotherapy
Jeffrey (1984)	Non-specific, 1984	Assess cost of chemotherapy in PHC	Chloroquine
Kaewsonthi and Harding (1984)	Thailand, 2 zones, pop. 1 m and 0.5 m, 1980–1	Assess cost and performance of surveillance	Case detection and treatment activities
Kaewsonthi (1988)	Thailand, 2 zones	As above	As above
MacCormack et al. (1989)	The Gambia	Assess impregnated bednets	Impregnated and non-impregnated bednets; chemoprophylaxis
Mills (1990)	Nepal, national programme and sample of districts, 1983 and 1984	Assess cost and effectiveness of routine control programme	Vector control; case detection and treatment
Molineaux and Gramiccia (1980)	Garki district, Kano State, Nigeria, 1969–79	Assess effectiveness of control measures	Various combinations of insecticide; mass drug administration; larviciding
Nevill et al. (1988)	Kenyan school	Assess effectiveness	Bednets; chemoprophylaxis
Ortiz (1968)	Paraguay, 1965–72, national programme	Projection of cost of eradication programme	Insecticides; case detection and treatment
Phillips and Mills (1991)	Nepal, 1986, national programme	Compare operational costs of insecticides	Insecticides: DDT, malathion, bendiocarb
Sharma (1986)	Kheda district, Gujerat, India, 1985	Compare chemical and environmental control methods	Spraying with DDT and malathion; environmental management
Smith (1985)	Non-specific	Assess cost per capita	DDT spraying; surveillance
Sudre and MacFarlane (1990)	Africa	Assess treatment of chloroquine resistant malaria in children	Treatment
Walsh and Warren (1979)	Non-specific	Identify priority primary health care interventions	Vector control

Table 4 Cost-effectiveness ratios of malaria control projects (US$, 1984)

Country	Control method	Annual cost per person protected	Cost per case prevented[a]	Cost per death averted	Reference
LDCs	Drugs	0.07[b]	—	—	Bruce-Chwatt (1987)
LDCs	Drugs	0.07[b]	—	—	Jeffrey (1984)
Taiwan	Surveillance	0.10	—	—	Griffith (1961)
Thailand	Case detection and treatment	0.13 and 0.25	—	—	Kaewsonthi (1988)
Thailand	Case detection and treatment, vector control	0.16 and 0.61	—	—	Kaewsonthi and Harding (1984)
India	Surveillance	0.19	—	—	Griffith (1961)
Nepal	Case detection and treatment[c]	0.19-0.60	2.40-68.50	119-11 938	Mills (1990)
Thailand	Surveillance	0.20	—	—	Griffith (1961)
Thailand	Spraying	0.20	—	—	Griffith (1961)
Taiwan	Combined methods	0.26	—	—	Griffith (1961)
India (Kheda)	Environmental management	0.27	—	—	Sharma (1986)
India (national programme)	Spraying and surveillance	0.29	—	—	Griffith (1961)
Nepal	Spraying	0.39	—	—	Griffith (1961)
Nepal	Combined methods[c]	0.37-0.60	1.52-154.46	74-12 034	Mills (1990)
Thailand	Vector control	0.40 and 0.41	—	—	Kaewsonthi (1988)
Greece	Surveillance	0.41	—	—	Griffith (1961)
Indonesia	Spraying	0.42	—	—	Griffith (1961)
Ceylon	Spraying and surveillance	0.43	—	—	Griffith (1961)
Taiwan	Spraying	0.43	—	—	Griffith (1961)
Indonesia	Spraying and	0.49	—	—	Griffith (1961)

Country	Method				Reference
Taiwan	Spraying	0.43	—	—	Griffith (1961)
Indonesia	Spraying and surveillance	0.49	—	—	Griffith (1961)
Nepal	Spraying[c]	0.61–1.91	—	—	Mills (1990)
India (Kheda)	Spraying	0.63	—	—	Sharma (1986)
Sudan	Spraying	0.75	—	—	El Gaddal et al. (1985)
The Gambia	Impregnated bednets, chemoprophylaxis for children	1.09	—	—	MacCormack et al. (1989)
Taiwan	Spraying and surveillance	1.25	—	—	Griffith (1961)
LDCs	Surveillance, spraying	1.47	—	—	Smith (1985)
Indonesia	Vector control	1.57 and 4.85	75.00 and 92.10	—	Gandahusada et al. (1984)
Nigeria (Sokoto)	Spraying	1.63	—	—	Bruce-Chwatt and Archibald (1959)
Kenya	Bednets	1.66	—	—	Nevill et al. (1988)
LDCs	Vector control	2.97	—	892.20	Walsh and Warren (1979)
Liberia	Case detection and treatment, vector control	6.64	12.30	—	Hedman et al. (1979)
India	Vector control	—	1.88	—	Cohn (1973)
Paraguay	Vector control	—	53.77	—	Ortiz (1968)
Nigeria (Garki)	Case detection and treatment, vector control	—	233.15	—	Molineaux and Gramiccia (1980)
Sri Lanka	Vector control	—	—	69.95	Barlow (1968)

Source: Barlow and Grobar (1985); references cited in table.
[a] Annual costs divided by annual number of cases (deaths) prevented, or total cost during project life divided by number of case-years (deaths) prevented during project life.
[b] Drug costs only.
[c] The cost range encompasses (1) areas of different endemicity and (2) different assumptions on cases and deaths prevented.

Most studies are concerned with choices of *preventive* strategies. Within this heading, little attention has been paid to the choice between alternative case detection and treatment methods, with a few exceptions. Of these, the most comprehensive studies are those of Kaewsonthi (1988) and Mills (1990), which both undertook an extensive comparison of case detection and treatment methods. Mills (1990) included in the comparison all the other strategies of the Nepalese malaria control programme. In both studies, absence of good epidemiological data forced the authors to rely heavily on intermediate effectiveness measures (e.g. cases detected). A few other strategies aimed at the individual have been evaluated in economic terms such as bednets (Schreck and Self, 1985; MacCormack *et al.*, 1989), but so far with only partial cost or effectiveness information.

Most attention has been directed to preventive measures aimed at the environment. The use of residual insecticides has been extensively evaluated in terms of their insecticidal properties, safety, and required dosages and frequency of application. Rarely, however, do such studies consider their impact on the incidence of malaria or their cost over and above that of the insecticide alone. Exceptions are the study by Gandahusada *et al.* (1984) of fenitrothion and by Phillips and Mills (1991) of the operational (delivery) costs of DDT, malathion and bendiocarb.

Although the provision of *diagnosis and treatment* often absorbs substantial resources, little attention has been paid to the costs of alternative patterns of provision of routine treatment services. Several studies have estimated the cost of including chemotherapy for malaria in primary health care (e.g. Jeffrey, 1984) and an interesting study evaluates the cost implications of microscopy prior to treatment and of alternatives to chloroquine (Schapira, 1989).

Given the importance of malaria control in the health budgets of many countries, it seems surprising to conclude from this summary that only two studies, those by Kaewsonthi and Harding (1984) and Kaewsonthi (1988) and by Mills (1989, 1990), have begun to explore the innumerable choices concerning the strategies and organization of malaria control. The dearth of reliable data and the different circumstances in which studies have been conducted make it difficult to conclude from Table 4 that one malaria control strategy (or a particular mix) is unquestionably superior to another. That said, some tentative conclusions can be drawn.

It is interesting to note that the costs found by Griffith (1961) are not very different from more recent estimates for national programmes using combined strategies (e.g. Thailand and Nepal). As might be expected, however, recent vector control costs, expressed per capita of the population protected, are considerably higher than their 1960s counterparts, reflecting both the increased cost of insecticides and a switch to more expensive insecticides.

The ratio 'cost per case prevented' is difficult to interpret because it can be influenced by many factors. The higher the initial incidence, the greater will be the potential reduction in incidence on application of a control measure. This fact helps to account, for instance, for the very low cost per case prevented in India and per death prevented in Sri Lanka. Other influences will be the characteristics of the vector and environment as expressed in the basic case reproduction rate (helping to account for the high cost in the Garki project, Nigeria, where control measures had to be applied intensively to be effective) and population density (helping to account for the relatively cheap control in the Liberian project where a mining town was the location of control efforts).

A few of the studies listed in Table 4 shed light on the choice of strategy. In terms of cost per person protected, spraying is far more expensive than case detection and treatment, implying that its effectiveness would have to be far greater for it to be cost-effective, though the more expensive the insecticide, the greater the potential for reducing costs by selective coverage (Mills, 1989). In terms of case detection and treatment method, both Kaewsonthi and Mills found that the cost per case detected through an active method was much greater than that of passive methods, and that malaria clinics were a relatively cheap means of detecting and treating cases. Mills also found that the desirability of the integration of malaria control with general health services depended partly on the level of malaria: while case detection and treatment was much cheaper in districts with integrated services at low levels of malaria, their costs were likely to approach those of vertically organized districts as cases rose.

With the current interest in impregnated bednets, more studies are required of their cost-effectiveness in different circumstances. It seems they can be a relatively cheap and effective source of protection in The Gambia (MacCormack et al., 1989). However, in Nepal their cost per capita was much higher than that of other control methods (Mills, 1989).

Cost-effectiveness studies of vector control through environmental management have shown it to be cost-effective for vector control in many circumstances in the USA (PEEM, 1986). Whether this conclusion applies elsewhere is uncertain; the value of environmental management is likely to be site-specific, depending on the vector, nature of the environment and size and location of breeding sites, and on the degree of malarial endemicity.

Gaps in knowledge

In summary, a number of topics stand out as requiring immediate attention:
(1) How do individuals view the danger of malaria and how do they respond to it? What are the determinants of demand for public and private sector treatment? Can this demand be influenced — e.g. by information campaigns, subsidies for purchases of bednets?
(2) What is the cost-effectiveness of existing malaria control strategies, both singly and in combination and at different levels of output?
(3) In countries where there is no organized control effort, is investment in

malaria control likely to bring greater returns in terms of health than investment in other currently neglected health programmes?

(4) What is the appropriate role of the private sector in financing (e.g. direct payments by individuals) and provision (e.g. sale of drugs and bednets)?

Malaria vaccines: thoughts for the future?

If a safe and efficacious vaccine becomes available, a series of economic decisions will have to be taken.

First, the most appropriate time for an economic evaluation must be identified. There is little point in doing a study before a vaccine is shown to be effective and safe. However, the pressure to use a proven vaccine is likely to be very great, so an economic evaluation must be done as early as possible.

Secondly, detailed consideration must be given to the innumerable choices concerning the use of the vaccine. The history of technological innovation shows that diffusion often simply happens, on a much more widespread basis than intended, and with little rationale for the way in which a new technology is used (viz. CT scanners). It is now generally agreed (Culyer and Horisberger, 1983) that planning guidelines are required for any new technology to indicate the most cost-effective patterns of use. The main choices to be evaluated are those indicated in Figure 2 and discussed below.

Choice of delivery strategy

For example, should the vaccine be delivered on its own, or integrated in routine immunization or general health services? Much will depend on the age-group targeted and the coverage sought. Integration with an EPI programme is likely to be cost-effective if the vaccine can be delivered at the same time as other vaccines: however, older children and adults will need to be reached in other ways. Delivery of vaccine through a special programme may be seen as an attractive option in the short term in order to achieve high coverage: it is unlikely to be a cost-effective strategy in the long run.

Choice of target group

If the vaccine is very expensive, it may be cost-effective only for high-risk groups or individuals. Any economic evaluation must therefore include consideration of target groups (and the costs of identifying them if they are not easily accessible).

Choice of place of intervention

A malaria vaccine could be delivered at home (or nearby in the village) or at a health facility. The choice between them, or the relative emphasis to be given to each, will depend on the costs of each and the coverage sought. Vaccination at a health facility is likely to be cheap but coverage will be limited, at least of older children and adults. Whether the extra cost of outreach is considered worthwhile will depend on the value placed on increased coverage. This itself will in part depend on whether interruption of transmission can be expected at a coverage level achievable by outreach.

Choice of time of intervention

It is likely that choices will exist on when to give the vaccine to young children, and how frequently it needs to be readministered to children and adults. These choices are likely to involve a trade-off between increased cost and increased protection. They will be very difficult to make because of uncertainties in the early years of vaccine use about the length of the protective effect.

Once the most efficient pattern of use of the vaccine has been identified, the costs per case and death prevented by the vaccine must be compared with those of other malaria control strategies. It is quite possible that in the circumstances of some countries a vaccine may be effective but not economically efficient (alternative uses of the resources would bring greater returns). This assessment will be helped if the economic evaluation includes a sensitivity analysis so that it is possible to assess how its conclusions might change if the values of particular variables differ (e.g. if staff costs are higher relative to vaccine costs). The economic evaluation should also clearly identify the non-vaccine costs, so that if countries are offered the vaccine free, they have a starting point to assess the cost implications for their services. Finally, the comparison of malaria control strategies should include all costs, irrespective of whether they fall on the government or households, to ensure that decisions do not ignore the costs imposed on households.

Acknowledgement

I am most grateful for the careful scrutiny by John Picard of an earlier draft. The review reported here forms part of the work of the ODA–supported Health Economics and Financing Programme at the LSHTM.

References

Andreano R and Helminiak T (1988) Economics, health and tropical diseases. In Herrin AN and Rosenfield PL (eds) *Economics, Health and Tropical Diseases.* School of Economics, University of the Philippines
Audibert M (1986) Agricultural non-wage production and health status: a case-study in a tropical environment. *Journal of Development Economics, 24,* 275–291
Banguero H (1984) Socio-economic factors associated with malaria in Colombia. *Social Science and Medicine, 19,* 1099–1104
Barlow R (1967) The effects of malaria eradication. *American Economic Review,* May, 130–148

Barlow R (1968) *The Economic Effects of Malaria Eradication*. Bureau of Public Health Economics, University of Michigan, Ann Arbor

Barlow R and Grobar LM (1985) *Cost and Benefits of Controlling Parasitic Diseases*. PHN Technical Note 85-17, Population, Health and Nutrition Department, World Bank, Washington DC

Behrman R and Deolikar AB (1988) Health and nutrition. In Chenery H and Srinivasan TN (eds) *Handbook of Development Economics*. Amsterdam, North-Holland

Bhombore SR, Brooke-Worth C and Nanjundiah KS (1952) A survey of the economic status of villagers in a malarial irrigated tract in Mysore State, India. *Indian Journal of Malariology*, *6*, 355–365

Birdsall N (1990) Health and development: what can research contribute? Forthcoming in (untitled) book of proceedings of workshop on contribution of social science research to health transition, Chen, LC *et al.* (eds)

Bonilla de Castro E (1985) Development of research training project in socio-economics of malaria eradication in Colombia, executive summary. Unpublished report to Special Programme for Research and Training in Tropical Diseases, WHO, Geneva

Brohult J, Jorfeldt L, Rombo L, Björkman A, Pehrson P-O, Sirleaf V and Bengtsson E (1981) The working capacity of Liberian males: a comparison between urban and rural populations in relation to malaria. *Annals of Tropical Medicine and Parasitology*, *75*, 487–494

Bruce-Chwatt LJ (1963) A longitudinal survey of natural malaria infection in a group of West African adults. *West African Medical Journal*, *12*, 141–173, 199–217

Bruce-Chwatt LJ (1987) Malaria and its control: present situation and future prospects. *Annual Review of Public Health*, *8*, 75–110

Bruce-Chwatt LJ and Archibald HM (1959) Malaria control project in Western Sokoto, Northern Nigeria: a report on four years results. *Proceedings of the 6th International Congress of Tropical Medicine and Malaria*, *7*, 347–361

Castro EB and Mokate KM (1988) Malaria and its socio-economic meanings: the study of Cunday in Colombia. In Herrin AN and Rosenfield PL (eds) *Economics, Health and Tropical Diseases*, School of Economics, University of the Philippines

Chernin E (1954) Problems in tropical public health among workers at a jute mill near Calcutta. 1. Malaria in the labour population. *American Journal of Tropical Medicine and Hygiene*, *31*, 74–93

Cohn EJ (1973) Assessing the costs and benefits of anti-malaria programmes: the Indian experience. *American Journal of Public Health*, *63*, 1086–1096

Conly GN (1975) *The Impact of Malaria on Economic Development: A Case Study*. Pan American Health Organization Scientific Publication no. 297, Washington DC

Culyer AJ and Horisberger B (eds) (1983) *Economic and Medical Evaluation of Health Care Technologies*. Springer-Verlag, Berlin

Drummond MF and Mills A (1987) *Survey of Cost-effectiveness and Cost–Benefit Analyses of Key Primary Health Care Projects in Commonwealth Countries*. Commonwealth Secretariat, London

El Gaddal AA, Haridi AAM, Hassan FT and Husein H (1985) Malaria control in the Gazira-Managil irrigated scheme of the Sudan. *Journal of Tropical Medicine and Hygiene*, *88*, 153–159

Ettling MB, Thimasarn K, Krachaiklin S and Bualoubai P (1989) Evaluation of malaria clinics in Maesot, Thailand: use of serology to assess coverage. *Transactions of the Royal Society of Tropical Medicine and Hygiene*, *83*, 325–331

Fernandez RE and Sawyer DO (1988) Socio-economic and environmental factors affecting malaria in an Amazon frontier area. In Herrin AN and Rosenfield PL (eds) *Economics, Health and Tropical Diseases*. School of Economics, University of the Philippines

Fungladda W, Sormani S, Klongkaunuankarn K and Hungsapruek (1987) Sociodemographic and behavioural factors associated with hospital malaria patients in Kanchanaburi, Thailand. *Journal of Tropical Medicine and Hygiene*, 90, 233–237

Gandahusada S, Fleming GA, Sukauto DT, Suwarto SN, Bang IH, Arwati S and Arit H (1984) Malaria control with residual fenitrothion in Central Java, Indonesia: an operational-scale trial using both full and selective coverage treatments. *Bulletin of the World Health Organization*, 62, 783–794

Gazin P, Freier C, Turk P, Sineste B and Carnevale P (1988) Le paludisme chez les employés d'une entreprise industrielle africaine. *Annales de la Société Belge de Médecine Tropicale*, 68, 285–292

Ghana Health Assessment Project Team (1981) A quantitative method of assessing the health impact of different diseases in less developed countries. *International Journal of Epidemiology*, 10, 73–80

Goldschmidt-Clermont L (1987) *Economic Evaluation of Unpaid Household Work: Africa, Asia, Latin America and Oceania*. Women, Work and Development no. 14, ILO, Geneva

Griffith DHS, Ramara DV and Mashaal H (1971) Contribution of health to development. *International Journal of Health Services*, 1, 253–318

Griffith ME (1961) Financial implications of surveillance in India and other countries. *Bulletin of the National Society of India for Malaria and other mosquito-borne diseases*, 9, 385–411

Guyer R and Candy D (1979) Injectable antimalaria therapy in tropical Africa: iatrogenic disease and wasted medical resources. *Transactions of the Royal Society of Tropical Medicine and Hygiene*, 73, 230–232

Hall SA and Wilks NE (1967) A trial of chloroquine-medicated salt for malaria suppression in Uganda. *American Journal of Tropical Medicine and Hygiene*, 16, 429–442

Hedman P, Brohult J, Forslund J, Sirleat V and Bengtsson F (1979) A pocket of controlled malaria in a holoendemic region of West Africa. *Annals of Tropical Medicine and Parasitology*, 73, 317–325

Herrin AN and Rosenfield PL (1988) *Economics, Health and Tropical Diseases*. School of Economics, University of the Philippines

Jamison DT and Mosley WH (forthcoming) Selecting disease control priorities in developing countries. In Jamison DT and Mosley WH (eds) *Disease Control Priorities in Developing Countries*. World Bank, Washington DC

Jeffrey G (1984) The role of chemotherapy in malaria control through primary health care: constraints and future prospects. *Bulletin of the World Health Organization*, 62, (Suppl.) 349–353.

Kaewsonthi S (1988) *Internal and External Costs of Malaria Surveillance in Thailand*. Social and Economic Research Report no. 6, TDR, WHO, Geneva

Kaewsonthi S and Harding AG (1984) Cost and performance of malaria surveillance in Thailand. *Social Science and Medicine*, 19, 1081–1097

Khan MJ (1966) Estimate of economic loss due to malaria in West Pakistan. *Pakistan Journal of Health*, 16, 187–193

Klarman HE (1979) Health economics and health economics research. *Milbank Memorial Fund Quarterly Bulletin*, 57, 371–379

Kuhner A (1971) The impact of public health programmes on economic development: report of a study of malaria in Thailand. *International Journal of Health Services*, 1, 285–292

Lee K and Mills A (1985) *The Economics of Health in Developing Countries*. Oxford University Press

Livadas SA and Athanassatos D (1963) The economic benefits of malaria eradication in Greece. *Rivista di Malariologia*, 42, 177–187

MacCormack CP, Snow RW and Greenwood BM (1989) Use of insecticide-impregnated bed nets in Gambian primary health care: economic aspects. *Bulletin of the World Health Organization, 67*, 209–214

Mason J and Hobbs J (1977) Malaria field studies in a high-incidence coastal area of El Salvador, C.A. *Bulletin of the Pan American Health Organization, 11*, 17–30

Miller MJ (1958) Observations on the natural history of malaria in the semi-resistant West African. *Transactions of the Royal Society of Tropical Medicine and Hygiene, 52*, 152–168

Mills A (1989) The application of cost-effectiveness analysis to disease control programmes in developing countries, with special reference to malaria control in Nepal. PhD thesis, University of London

Mills A (1990) *The Economic Evaluation of Malaria Control Technologies: The Case of Nepal.* Paper presented to the Second World Conference on Health Economics, Zurich, 10–14 September, 1990 (forthcoming in *Social Science and Medicine*)

Mills A (forthcoming) The impact of malaria on the economic development of Nepal. In Lee K and Mills A (eds) *Health Economics Research in Developing Countries.* Oxford University Press

Molineaux L and Gramiccia G (1980) *The Garki Project: Research on the Epidemiology and Control of Malaria in the Sudan Savanna of West Africa.* World Health Organization, Geneva

Nevill CG, Watkins WM, Caster JI and Munatu CG (1988) Comparison of mosquito nets, proguanil hydrochloride and placebo to prevent malaria. *British Medical Journal, 297*, 401–403

Niazi AD (1969) Approximate estimates of the economic loss caused by malaria with some estimates of the benefits of MEP in Iraq. *Bulletin of Endemic Diseases, II*, 28–39

Nur ETM and Mahran HA (1988) The effect of health on agricultural labour supply: a theoretical and empirical investigation. In Herrin AN and Rosenfield PL (eds) *Economics, Health and Tropical Diseases.* School of Economics, University of the Philippines

Ortiz JR (1968) Estimate of the cost of a malaria eradication programme. *Bulletin of the Pan American Health Organization*, 14–17

PEEM (Panel of Experts on Environmental Management for Vector Control) (1986) *Report of the sixth meeting.* VBF/86.2, PEEM Secretariat, World Health Organization, Geneva

Quo WK (1959) In World Health Organization, Malaria information. Unpublished working document. World Health Organization: Mal/Inform/46

Pehrson PO, Björkman A, Brohult J, Jorfeldt L, Lundbergh P, Rombo L, Willcox M and Bengtsson E (1984) Is the working capacity of Liberian industrial workers increased by regular malaria prophylaxis? *Annals of Tropical Medicine and Parasitology, 78*, 453–458

Phillips M and Mills A (1991) The operational costs of spraying residual insecticides: a case-study from Nepal. *Journal of Tropical Medicine and Hygiene, 94*, 130–139

Phillips M, Mills A and Dye C (forthcoming) *Cost-effectiveness Analysis of Vector Control Interventions: Guidelines for Water-resource Development Staff and Vector-borne Disease Programme Managers.* Joint WHO/FAO/UNEP Panel of Experts on Environmental Management for Vector Control

Picard J and Mills A (1990) The effects of malaria on the work time of different socio-economic groups: analysis of data from two Nepali districts. Health Policy Unit, London School of Hygiene and Tropical Medicine

Rajagopalan PK and Panicker KN (1985) Financial rewards ensure community involvement. *World Health Forum, 6*, 174–176

Ramaiah TJ (1980) *Cost–Benefit Analysis of Malaria Control and Eradication Pro-*

grammes in India. Public Systems Group, Indian Institute of Management, Ahmedabad

Rao CSN and Bhombore SR (1956) A survey of the economic status of villages in a malarious tract in Mysore State (India) after residual insecticidal spraying. *Bulletin of the National Society of India for Malaria and other mosquito-borne diseases*, 4, 71–77

Rosenthal G (1979) Of economists and economics, ceteris paribus. *Milbank Memorial Fund Quarterly Bulletin*, 57, 291–296

Ruberu PS (1977) Economic justification of intensive malaria control programme in Sri Lanka 1977/81. Unpublished

Ruebush II TK, Goday-Bonilla HA and Klein RE (1985) Improving malaria detection by volunteer workers. *World Health Forum*, 6, 274–277

Russell PF and Menon MK (1942) A malario-economic survey in rural South India. *Indian Medical Gazette*, 77, 167–180

Samuelson PA (1976) *Economics*, 10th edn. McGraw-Hill, New York

San Pedro C (1967–8) Economic costs and benefits of malaria eradication. *Philippines Journal of Public Health*, 12, 5–24

Schapira A (1989) Chloroquine resistant malaria in Africa: the challenge to health services. *Health Policy and Planning*, 4, 17–28

Schreck CE and Self LS (1985) Bed nets that kill mosquitos. *World Health Forum*, 63, 342–344

Sharma VP (1986) *Cost-effectiveness of Environmental Management for Malaria Control in India*. Working paper prepared for 6th meeting of the Panel of Experts on Environmental Management for Vector Control, Geneva, 8–12 September

Shepard DS, Brinkmann U, Ettling MB and Sauerborn R (1990) *Economic Impact of Malaria in Africa*. Vector Biology and Control Project, Arlington, Virginia

Sinton JA (1935–6) What malaria costs India nationally, socially and economically. *Records of the Malaria Survey of India*, 5, 223–264, 413–489; 6, 96–169

Smith A (1985) *Cost Implications of Insecticide Resistance in Vector Control*. VBC/ECV/85.20, WHO, Geneva

Sudan, Democratic Republic of (1975) *National Health Programme 1977/8–1983/4*. Khartoum, Government Printing Office

Sudre P and MacFarlane D (1990) Treatment of chloroquine resistant malaria in African children: a cost-effectiveness analysis. CDC, US Department of Health, and Human Service.

Van Dine DL (1916) The relation of malaria to crop production. *Scientific Monthly*, November, 431–439

Vosti S (1990) Malaria among gold miners in Southern Para, Brazil: estimates of determinants and individual costs. *Social Science and Medicine*, 30, 1097–1105

Walsh JA and Warren KS (1979) Selective primary health care: an interim strategy for disease control in developing countries. *New England Journal of Medicine*, 301, 967–974

Wright J (1977) An economic analysis of malaria control in Java–Bali–Madura and Outer Islands. Unpublished

WORKSHOP REPORT AND RECOMMENDATIONS
RAPPORTEUR: SOMKID KAEWSONTHI

Little is known about the economics of malaria control, and there are uncertainties about what has been reported, leaving what Mills has called 'gaps in our knowledge'.

Given this situation, four important questions should be addressed:

(1) What, if any, are the recommendations for action (not research) which can be derived from previous research findings?
(2) What should be the basis for deciding the research agenda to support current control operations?
(3) What should be the priorities in that research agenda?
(4) When should economic analysis of vaccine delivery be undertaken and what will be the objectives and priorities?

Actions from past research?

With few exceptions, little action has or could be derived from existing research findings.

It is somewhat surprising that control activities were not more clearly driven by economic considerations even though the costs and effectiveness of services would be influenced by the mix of services and the local context. Four factors contribute to this situation:

(1) Few studies have been undertaken.
(2) Knowledge of costs and effectiveness did not of themselves produce changes in organizations particularly where there are long-established practices. The constraint was and is organizational rather than economic.
(3) To determine the costs and effectiveness of alternative mixes of services it is necessary to monitor costs and performance during changes.
(4) The costs and performance of services are only one side of the equation. These services also affect the costs to patients. Several studies have now reported on these aggregate costs.

Benefit–cost ratios based upon lost production are positive but the ratio depends upon what is included, on valuation and location. In Africa, where malaria is mainly a disease of children and expenditure on control is low, benefits in money value might be roughly equal to costs. But in other areas, such as South-East Asia, where the disease affects adults, benefits are significantly greater than costs even given labour substitution. Judgment of benefits in production/development/money terms is contentious and should not be the only goal. The welfare benefit from preventing infection and treating people who have malaria is a valid and readily quantifiable goal in itself.

Several non-economists criticized the uncharacteristic reluctance of the economists present to draw conclusions and make recommendations due to methodological uncertainties and/or the delicate relations with control organizations. Funding agencies urgently require advice on the costs of malaria and the benefit–cost ratio to be achieved through control. Such evidence is essential to support efforts to raise more funds for malaria research and control.

Given forty years of malaria eradication and control programmes one may well wonder what was the basis for past decisions to fund these programmes world-wide. Political? Humanitarian? Expectations or evidence that control of the disease would lead to faster economic development?

Criteria for defining the research agenda

Since economics appears to have made little contribution in the past to control operations, what then should be the criteria for deciding the future research agenda? The answer should not be 'gaps in our knowledge', interest or academic significance but confidence that the questions researched will result in improvements in the efficiency of control operations.

This means not only considering the questions to be studied, but also the techniques for data collection and analysis and the very process of research.

Research questions should be determined by those who would make the decisions so that the answers will be accepted and could affect the actions taken. At the micro level this means local answers to local problems since, as evidenced by moves to stratification, economic analyses may have little global validity outside the study area.

Techniques for data collection and analysis should be such that they can be used on a *regular basis* by local organizations with the resources they have available. And the research process must be with and through the control organization since only then may results be accepted and used.

The research agenda

What then are the issues of local and general concern?

(1) *Economic benefits.* If malaria control is accepted as a legitimate development objective in its own right then there is, in principle, no need to measure benefits in money terms. However, more should be known about the effect of malaria on schooling and education.

(2) *Interventions.* The use of cost/case as a measure of cost-effectiveness should be clarified since there are confusions in its use and it ignores scale.

Specific questions are how to identify the optimum mix and distribution of different types of services in a given context and how to measure costs and effectiveness, particularly in conjunction with epidemiology and clinical trial interventions.

(3) *Finance and organization.* Analysis of malaria control efficiency and arguments to support requests for more funding at the international level are hampered by a lack of information on the current level and recent trends in expenditure on malaria control. A study should be made of public and aggregate expenditure at regional and world level. At the micro level, where there are proposals for some move from public to private provider, studies are required to determine the pattern and determinants of malaria drug distribution and consumption through the private sector.

Many organizations which have provided a fixed menu of malaria control services for decades are gradually, if reluctantly, adopting changes in practice. These changes provide an opportunity and a need to analyse the economics of integration of services, integration of vector-borne disease control, and malaria control with PHC.

(4) *Methodological issues.* Methodological issues concern measures of efficiency and procedures for measuring costs and performance.

As a monitoring tool, cost per case detected suffers from two defects, namely an increase as the number of cases decreases, and a poor stimulus to improve the effectiveness of case detection. Efforts have been made to develop alternative measures which overcome these deficiencies: a model of the pool of infection (the number of man-days per year there are infective carriers in the community) and a case-prevented model (Kaewsonthi, 1989). Much more work needs to be done on this approach.

In terms of methodologies there are two concerns: first, to improve research methodologies so that programme managers can monitor their own costs and performance on a regular basis without too much effort; secondly, if required, to standardize cost–benefit studies so that comparison can be made of country studies and the findings generalized.

Malaria vaccine

Mills proposed that a series of economic decisions — how to deliver, who receives, where administered and when given — will have to be taken when vaccines become available. There was general agreement that the economics of field testing a vaccine should be undertaken now through modelling and 'what ... if' scenarios. The determinants of costs and significance of variables on costs would provide valuable information to funding agencies and vaccine manufacturers. Knowledge of costs will be essential when planning superimposition and/or substitution of vaccines for other treatments.

In economic terms, when and where to deliver a vaccine should be until marginal cost of delivery equals marginal benefit. However, in making the calculation, welfare objectives and the time-frame should be agreed. The marginal cost of eradicating the last cases of smallpox was very high. But the marginal benefit over future generations will be immense.

Reference

Kaewsonthi, S. (1989) Internal and external costs of malaria surveillance in Thailand. *Social and Economic Research Report No. 6*, TDR/WHO, Geneva

Organization of control

Awash Teklehaimanot

World Health Organization, Geneva, Switzerland

Introduction

The type of organization needed to undertake antimalaria activities depends very much on the size of the population at risk, the magnitude of the problem, the objectives of the programme and on the intervention methods and activities required to achieve them. Moreover, it is important to realize that the objectives, targets and strategies must be based on careful and detailed assessment of the overall socioeconomic situation of the country or area concerned and should be considered within the context of other equally pressing health needs and priorities. The technical and operational feasibility of adopting such strategies or undertaking activities, their affordability and their sustainability must be clearly determined at the outset. The following are some of the main factors for consideration:

- the socioeconomic impact of the disease and its public health importance as compared to other health problems or needs;
- the infrastructure and level of development of the general health services and their role in malaria control;
- the existence and development of specialized services for malaria control and their relationship with the general health services;
- the availability of trained manpower;
- the transport/communication/logistic facilities;
- the recognition by the communities concerned of the importance of malaria as their major health problem and their desire to control it;
- the availability and strength of community organization and a tradition of community participation;
- inter-sectoral collaboration of development agencies in the control of malaria;
- the national commitment for supporting the antimalaria activities on a long-term basis with respect to human and financial resources, policy and legal requirements.

Major types of organizational structures for antimalaria activities

Antimalaria activities in endemic countries are basically carried out through two major organizational structures: specialized services, mostly organized as vertical programmes, and the general health services system. The organizational structure needed will vary depending on whether the objective of the programme is eradication or control of malaria.

Objectives and organization for malaria eradication

The global malaria eradication programme, which was launched in 1955 and carried out until 1969, had as its objective 'the ending of transmission of malaria, the elimination of the reservoir of infective cases, and the prevention of the re-establishment of transmission' (WHO, 1957) within a time-frame of about four to eight years. This required a large organizational structure to undertake specific tasks needing full coverage, i.e. spraying of all houses, collection and microscopic examination of blood smears and determination of the origin of malaria infections through investigation and classification of cases. Since the emphasis was on the detection and elimination of all infection, an extensive network of active and passive case detection posts was established to screen and take blood smears from all fever cases in communities. The spraying activities were standardized and carried out in all malarious areas regardless of their epidemiological differences (WHO, 1961).

The extensive campaigns were launched through 'vertical organizations' which were established outside the framework of the general health services. Such organizations, by necessity, became exceedingly complex, labour-intensive and consumed a significant proportion of the total health budget. Next to the cost of insecticides, the single largest budget item was wages for the large workforce.

In spite of such efforts and relatively efficient organization, it was soon realized that global eradication was not attainable during the specified time period. It also became apparent that without strengthened and developed general health services, it was difficult to maintain whatever was achieved through the eradication campaign (WHO, 1962). As a result, the objective of global malaria eradication was abandoned and subsequently most of the eradication programmes were transformed into control programmes.

Malaria control through vertical programmes

In line with the objectives of control and with the adapted strategy of an integrated primary health care approach, many malaria-endemic countries have found it necessary to either streamline the existing eradication-based organizational structure or develop a system within the general health services for undertaking cost-effective control programmes. As a result, most of the vertical programmes have undergone a series of modifications in their organizational structure. The methods used to attain an integrated approach as well as the rates of progress towards this aim are variable, resulting in different 'mixtures' of vertical and integrated components.

In some countries the vertical malaria control programmes are still single-purpose. They function with their own lines of command, staff and supplies, from the centre to the periphery, alongside the general health services system. They provide services related to case management, transmission control and management of epidemics. Such vertical programmes are essentially in an eradication mode, laying strong emphasis on transmission control and assuming responsibility for diagnosis and treatment of malaria cases.

In other situations, some single-purpose vertical malaria control programmes have been reorganized to include other vector-borne diseases with a decentralized system of technical and managerial decision-making. The decentralization of laboratory services to extend down to the district and subdistrict levels has facilitated early diagnosis and treatment. Even in this type of vertical programme, the problems of case management, especially for severe and complicated cases, and of referral procedures through the general health services are not satisfactorily resolved.

In some countries, the vertical programmes have been physically integrated into the general health service, in terms of administration and finances but without any clear guidance or explicit arrangements for establishing job descriptions and defining the respective technical responsibilities for the various categories of the large malaria control staff as well as for the health workers in the different levels of the general health services. Integration efforts, which have not been accompanied by training and reorientation of single-purpose workers to assume responsibility for a broader range of tasks or by taking concrete steps to upgrade and develop the inadequate preventive programmes of the general health services, have resulted in the deterioration of services and the worsening of malaria situations.

In spite of the varied efforts to streamline the organization of the specialized services, many of the vertical malaria control programmes, remnants of eradication, still continue to carry out tasks using structures and concepts that had been specifically developed for eradication (Najera, 1989). Regular application of residual insecticides, active detection of cases through house-to-house visits, presumptive treatment of fever cases pending complete treatment on confirmation by microscopic examination, investigation of cases and the requirement of taking a blood smear from every fever case are tasks that are still being carried out by many control programmes. Such activities do not serve for prompt diagnosis and treatment but consume scarce resources which could be used in priority or problem areas. The spectrum of malaria control activities has already been analysed in detail in previous publications (Najera, 1989; Bruce-Chwatt, 1979).

Malaria control through the general health services

In some countries the decision that the general health services take on the responsibilities of malaria control was made as part of the policy for an integrated primary health care strategy. However, in most of these countries, the health services did not make the necessary arrangements for undertaking specialized activities such as vector control.

The general health services are limited by their inability to operate fully outside a health centre or hospital setting, and therefore may not be accessible to populations outside their immediate surroundings. This is particularly true of most African countries where the ratio of health facilities to the population size at risk is not favourable. In general, the infrastructure of the general health services focuses primarily on the provision of curative services, with minimum emphasis on preventive programmes.

In addition to the constraints of coverage, the existing infrastructure, orientation and training of the available health manpower of most of the general health services may not be adequate to contribute the specialized components of malaria control activities. These specialized components include: spraying of houses with residual insecticides; monitoring for the emergence and spread of resistance to antimalarial drugs and insecticides; monitoring of epidemiological, entomological, demographic and meteorological indicators for forecasting or early detection of epidemics; the need for immediate action to control epidemics that may require emergency preparedness, mass mobilization of personnel and material resources, and intervention measures related to vector control through spraying operations and to disease control through drug administration to large populations; undertaking operational research of relevance to malaria control; and carrying out special surveys and epidemiological analysis for trend assessment, evaluation of impact of intervention measures and for planning purposes.

Vertical versus integrated approach to malaria control

The operational difficulties within countries and the conceptual issues regarding the establishment of systems of health programmes and delivery through either a vertical or an integrated approach have been debated for some time (WHO, 1982). Since the organizational structure, including technical and managerial capability of the general health services, and the relative importance of vertical control services differ from country to country, it would not be realistic to come up with a single organizational arrangement applicable to all countries. Thus, appropriate country or area-specific arrangements should be elaborated by each malaria-endemic country striving towards an eventual integrated general health service with strong components of specialized programmes.

As part of such a process it will be important to re-examine some of the current activities of vertical programmes such as malarial disease management, which includes diagnosis and treatment, and vigilance of activities in malaria-free areas against possible introduction of cases and establishment of transmission. It is outside the competence and facilities of vertical programmes to deal with the management of severe and complicated malarial disease which may require hospitalization of the patient and treatment support. The problem of disease management is further complicated by the widespread and increasing prevalence of parasite resistance to drugs, a situation that will require special skills and training, potentially available only in the general health services. The deployment of single-purpose malaria control workers to monitor for the possible introduction of malaria into previously malaria-free areas is also an unnecessary duplication of effort. In addition to cost considerations, the assignment of such responsibilities to the general health services will enable the specialized services to concentrate instead on relevant activities in those areas where malaria is prevalent. Thus, the special programmes may need to be restructured to focus on vector control activities and other special tasks and relinquish disease management responsibilities to the general health services.

However, it is equally important to realize that the existing infrastructures and staffing patterns of most general health services are inadequate to undertake effective malaria control activities, particularly those related to transmission control and management of epidemics. Thus, the health services system needs restructuring to incorporate specialists on various aspects of malaria control, at least at the national level, who are qualified to develop control strategies and to provide technical guidance and supervision.

Ideal characteristics of malaria control organization

Whatever the arrangement, the services for malaria control need to be organized on administrative, financial and technical levels, with the necessary orientation and support to develop a decision-making capacity regarding the planning, implementation and evaluation of control activities at the local level. The following are some of the requirements for a cost-effective organizational structure:

• The availability of experts at the central and regional levels is a prerequisite for decentralization of services. The core of experts will be responsible for developing technical documents, evaluating the effectiveness of programme activities, validating the appropriate indicators and defining the minimum data requirements, as well as for providing the necessary support and guidance to regional and district health managers on various aspects of malaria control. Certain specialized activities and studies, such as determination of vector sensitivity to insecticides, will be carried out by the central or regional experts.

- The decentralized organizational set-up should be supported by an efficient referral system, a training component, operational research and an information system. The development of these facilities should be relevant to prevailing situations.
- The emphasis being on disease management, there should be clear and complete guidelines on diagnosis and treatment at all levels of the infrastructure.
- Because of the limited technical competence at the periphery and of problems of drug resistance, there is a need for establishing a system to ensure the recognition of treatment failures, the selection of appropriate drugs for use and also the monitoring of severe malaria case management. Therefore, decentralization of laboratory services towards the periphery is essential. A microscopic examination facility should be available, at least at the health centre level, and laboratory services need to be backed up by the necessary supplies, supervision and quality control.
- The availability of essential antimalarial drugs at all times and at all levels of the infrastructure is crucial to malaria control.
- The capability to determine the sensitivity of parasites to antimalarial drugs, using modified *in vivo* methods, should be developed, at least down to district level. However, all health personnel at all levels should be able to recognize treatment failures.
- The capability to analyse information collected at every level for immediate action is necessary. Monitoring for and timely recognition of epidemics is crucial for taking either preventive or control measures.
- The availability of health education materials on early diagnosis and treatment; treatment compliance; recognition, reporting and control of epidemics; and the role of personal and community-based protection measures against mosquito bites are important.
- Organized community participation in all aspects of malaria control is essential for success. It is important to use facilities that already exist in communities. School teachers, community leaders or traditional healers are some of the community assets that must be utilized.
- Once vector control measures appropriate for the local situation have been determined, intervention measures should have strong components of community participation and collaboration with other sectors.
- Appropriate plans and preparedness, in terms of establishing and maintaining reserves of sufficient drugs, insecticides and funds for the mobilization of health and other personnel and for other operational costs, should exist in the epidemic-prone areas or situations in order to facilitate timely control of epidemics.
- A mechanism for evaluating the impact of intervention measures should be part of the planning process.

Epidemiological bases for malaria control

The objectives of malaria control, as repeatedly stressed for many years, are 'the prevention/reduction of morbidity and mortality, the reduction of transmission whenever feasible and the prevention and control of epidemics' (WHO, 1979). The strategies required for achieving the objectives of malaria control are: management of the disease through the provision of early diagnosis and treatment; selective use of vector control measures; and management of epidemics through a combination of disease management practices and vector control measures. Implementation of these strategies requires a better understanding of the epidemiology of the disease.

The transmission of malaria and therefore the intensity of the problem is not uniformly distributed but rather varies from area to area, from season to season and from year to year. Some of the major causes for such focal distribution could be:

- differences in physical, ecological and social characteristics of an area and the population at risk;
- differential changes in meteorological conditions such as abnormal rainfall, temperature and humidity;
- introduction either of large non-immune population groups into malaria-endemic areas or of parasite carriers into potentially receptive areas;
- differences in vectorial capacity;
- creation of new foci of transmission as a result of man-made environmental changes related to exploitation of land for agriculture, timber industry, mining and other major development projects;
- regular application of insecticidal spraying aimed at reducing transmission may have as a 'side-effect' the lowering of immune status of communities. The populations of such communities are predisposed to increased risk whenever spraying activities are withdrawn.

As a result of this diversity of malaria situations, implementation of a set of control activities may not be effective everywhere. Recognizing that there is no universally applicable solution to the malaria problem, the principle of epidemiological stratification has been considered as an important tool for planning and implementing control activities targeted to any given country or area (WHO, 1986). This analytical approach has been based on the grouping of areas by epidemiological, entomological, demographic, climatological and other variables. However, this approach has often been constrained by the fact that many variables must be collected through special surveys, and by the absence of a generally accepted framework for linking strata with control options. Stratification in most cases has therefore not really guided malaria control efforts.

Major types of malaria paradigms

The weaknesses and constraints of the classical stratification approach have led to the development of a more pragmatic approach to epidemiological topologies. This approach involves the identification of a limited number of main ecological prototypes or paradigms based on accumulated empirical experience, their further characterization by local determinants, and the linkage between situations sharing certain characteristics and specific options for control. The following eight major paradigms currently identified are:

(1)   malaria of the African savanna;
(2)   forest malaria;
(3)   malaria associated with irrigated agriculture;
(4)   highland fringe malaria;
(5)   desert fringe and oasis malaria;
(6)   urban malaria;
(7)   settled agricultural communities;
(8)   coastal/marshland malaria.

Principal determinants

Each paradigm must be further characterized by epidemiological, operational and socioeconomic determinants. The following are some of the main determinants which may, to a greater or lesser extent, influence the principal features of each paradigm:

• population characteristics (immune status, movement and settlement patterns, socioeconomic and behavioural factors);
• level of endemicity/transmission (low to high endemicity, perennial, seasonal and epidemic transmission);
• the malaria parasite species involved and their susceptibility to antimalarial drugs;
• the anopheline vector species involved, their behaviour (breeding, feeding, resting) and their susceptibility to insecticides and the vector control practices taken on an individual and/or a community basis;
• the types and extent of development projects in the area (construction of dams, road building);
• the infrastructure of health services in place (government, non-governmental organizations, private practice).

By working through the relevant determinants for each of the paradigms empirically identified in a given country, it is possible to distil quickly the essence of a country's or area's malaria problem. Having identified and further characterized the nature of the problem, it will then be easier to develop appropriate control strategies and to select intervention tools. The management of malarial disease is fundamental to all malaria situations and must be undertaken irrespective of the type of paradigm. However, the paradigm approach will be useful for the identification of risk groups and priority areas (e.g. areas prone to epidemics and problems related to drug resistance) and the collection of other epidemiological information useful for the improvement of disease management practices. On the other hand, the subdivision of the problems into major paradigms and recognition of the variability of local epidemiological situations within each paradigm will facilitate the decision for selective use of vector control strategies appropriate to the particular epidemiological and ecological settings. Personal protective measures against vector mosquitoes (e.g. the use of repellents and bednets, improved housing, and the avoidance of outdoor activities during peak biting hours) should, however, be encouraged and supported in most situations.

One of the eight major paradigms, malaria associated with highland fringe, is briefly described as an illustration.

Highland fringe malaria

In general, there is no malaria transmission in highland areas, except in the lowest parts of their range adjacent to the malaria-endemic lowland areas and in isolated pockets where the microclimate and local physical characteristics are conducive to the breeding and survival of vector mosquitoes. The malaria problem is limited to these particular areas and therefore highland populations in general usually have a low level of immunity. Consequently, they are susceptible to infection when environmental conditions favour the vertical migration of vectors to the highland areas coupled with the introduction of reservoirs of infection. This will culminate in the occurrence of epidemics that have a potential for causing severe malaria in all age groups.

It is important to realize that the ecological conditions of highland areas are continuously modified by an overcrowded population involved in various activities, such as terracing of steep slopes, levelling of plains, and constructing water ponds. These activities are a means of overcoming the acute shortage of land for cultivation and the establishment of villages. These resulting changes are accompanied by an increasing trend for populations to move and to settle in the plains and in the modified areas at lower elevations. These events are of epidemiological importance as they lead to an increased potential for recurring epidemics over large areas and to possible increases in the size of the malaria transmission areas.

Malaria control activities in highland fringe areas

In highland fringe areas, where the risk of epidemics is high, it will be important to strengthen the health services' capacity to undertake early diagnosis and treatment and to establish mechanisms for monitoring key environmental (abnormal rainfall, temperature, humidity), entomological (vector density and longevity), clinical (morbidity and mortality rates), and demographic (population influx, drug consumption) indicators for alerting authorities of an impending new epidemic. It will also be necessary to develop a contingency plan to permit including the immediate availability of necessary resources and to facilitate rapid distribution of drugs and insecticides in the event of epidemics.

The control of a malaria epidemic involves relieving the immediate clinical consequences and preventing the spread of the epidemic through early diagnosis and treatment and intradomiciliary application of residual insecticides. This means improving disease management by strengthening the capacity for early diagnosis and for delivering effective treatment, with special emphasis on the management of severe cases. This requires an adequate supply of both antimalarial drugs and insecticides and a rapid capability to check the response of *Plasmodium falciparum* infected cases to the available antimalarial drugs and the susceptibility of malaria vectors to insecticides.

Timely application of intradomiciliary residual insecticide is also recommended to contain and control epidemics. However, residual insecticide spraying should be timed to the inter-epidemic period. Monitoring of key environmental, entomological and demographic indicators will be essential for timing the spraying operations.

In certain conditions, it may be necessary to supplement spraying operations with periodic mass drug administration using a combination of schizontocidal and gametocytocidal drugs. However, if the prevalence of chloroquine-resistant *P. falciparum* is fairly widespread, it becomes more difficult to find an acceptable regime for mass drug administration, given the risk of side-effects and of accelerating the development of resistance to alternative drugs. Mass chemoprophylaxis targeted to the most vulnerable groups, particularly new settlers, temporary workers, or populations in areas that are subjected to recent ecological changes favourable for mosquito breeding, may be appropriate before or during the epidemic.

References

Bruce-Chwatt LJ (1979) Man against malaria: conquest or defeat. *Transactions of the Royal Society of Tropical Medicine and Hygiene*, 73, 605–617

Najera JA (1989) Update: malaria and the work of WHO. *Bulletin of the World Health Organization, 67*, 229–243

WHO (1957) *Technical Report Series*, 123 (Malaria: Sixth report of the Expert Committee)

WHO (1961) *Technical Report Series*, 205 (Malaria: Eighth report of the Expert Committee)

World Health Assembly resolution (1962) WHA15.19

WHO (1979) *Technical Report Series*, 640 (WHO Expert Committee on Malaria: Seventeenth report)

WHO (1986) *Technical Report Series*, 735 (WHO Expert Committee on Malaria: Eighteenth report)
WHO (1982) *Technical Report Series*, 680 (Malaria control as part of primary health care)

WORKSHOP REPORT AND RECOMMENDATIONS
RAPPORTEUR: MARCEL TANNER

Organization of control here involves all aspects of the establishment, implementation and evaluation of malaria control activities in a given endemic setting, ranging from the technical aspects of making an epidemiological assessment to the management issues at national and district levels. Only general guidelines and checklists can be provided here for use by national and district health planners when preparing or reviewing malaria control activities without the opportunity to look at and evaluate experience in any particular country.

The chapter by Awash Teklehaimanot contrasted the vertical organization of malaria control with the organization of control within general services. These two concepts should be considered as the margins between which we have to place our organization of control in a given setting with its epidemiological, social, economic and political features.

The WHO strategic framework, which includes (1) community participation, (2) primary health care (PHC) principles, (3) health systems and operational research, and (4) the epidemiological paradigms for the classification of malaria endemic areas, should serve as the context within which control approaches should be planned and implemented.

It is important to pursue the epidemiological paradigm approach in order to classify malaria in any given country. This approach entails establishing a set of criteria, but still offers the possibility of flexibility, i.e. the addition of new paradigms once they become evident when a particular endemic setting is assessed. A possible risk of introducing the paradigm approach is that a country may be tempted to launch a major epidemiological and social science data collection exercise. Therefore, reaching a conclusion on any paradigm must be based chiefly on (1) existing data, (2) short site visits that include talks with community members and (3) mainly common sense.

Once the paradigms are established for a given setting, there are a number of prerequisites, discussed below, that must still be fulfilled *before* control objectives and strategies can be formulated.

An understanding of the communities involved

Too little attention is usually paid to the actual consumers of the control programme, and few control planners and managers talk (or know how to talk) to the communities concerned. Thus, before major activities are launched, communication with the communities needs to be well established, and steps in which the community will participate must be discussed and agreed upon.

Local priorities must be understood

Communication with the communities concerned and with the *local* authorities (political, social, cultural) should form the basis for identifying the position of malaria within the spectrum of all prevailing health and community development problems. This clearly involves understanding demand and the major determinants of health, disease and health-seeking behaviour in a community.

The level of commitment and support

Clarification of the first two prerequisites will automatically lead to an understanding of the degree of political will prevailing in a setting. The will expressed, however, needs to be contrasted with the support actually being provided by national and international authorities and funding bodies. In the past malaria control issues have contributed to the generation of PHC principles and guidelines, but, on the other hand, malaria control hardly receives any major support within existing PHC programmes, as is evidenced by funding patterns as well as by the position of malaria control within the PHC guidelines of many countries.

Once these three prerequisites have been established, they will provide the context in which control objectives can and should be formulated for any country/setting. This formulation step must also involve a critical assessment of the presently available control tools, with regard to the feasibility and affordability of applying them within a particular paradigm in a particular setting. It is at this level that technical *and* economic considerations, particularly concerning effectiveness, are required. Finally, establishing the prerequisites implies a substantial input from social scientists as well as from experts in biomedical sciences, malariology and health planning.

Once objectives have been formulated on the sound basis of the prerequisites mentioned, and in relation to the most effective tools, strategies will have to be selected. At this level, considering the extent to which the prerequisites have been fulfilled, and the objectives and strategies emerging from the local context, a national plan of control can be formulated.

The selection of strategies is a process that is strongly linked to the prevailing conditions in each setting/country. This summary can therefore only point to major determinants and elements to consider, rather than providing prescriptions or complete 'tool-boxes' for a country or a district.

Systems

Existing services need to be considered first, as the cornerstones of control operations. Existing services include not only the governmental health sector, but also NGOs, the private health sector and all other services related to health. Applying this broad definition may help to ensure that inter-sectoral collaboration will be firmly rooted at the strategic level and not only reflected at the conceptual or the operational level. Existing services need to be examined particularly for their staffing pattern, staff needs and requirements for staff training, both formal and (mainly) in-service, as well as for their ability to ensure the regular supply and rational use of drugs.

PHC and integration of malaria control into PHC are a vital part of the discussions on existing services. The organization of control in a given area will need to adhere to PHC principles. However, any plan for country or region should be oriented towards the level that its existing health care delivery services have actually reached, in relation to *national* PHC guidelines/policies. The orientation of malaria control by global PHC concepts can mislead planners, and divert a control programme away from national needs and demands.

Decentralization is a key issue for the management of the health care delivery services and therefore also for the organization of malaria control. For this to succeed, however, there is one basic principle: whenever a control organization does decentralize responsibility (technical and managerial), this step needs to be accompanied by a decentralization of authority. Decentralization very often fails because functions alone, but not the decision-making power, are shifted to peripheral levels.

Monitoring and evaluation are key elements of any disease control operation. There is a need to integrate most elements of the monitoring and evaluation process into existing services, in order to assure regional feedback and use of the information gathered. Monitoring and evaluation need to accompany all steps of control operations in order to ensure that the process of management control allows continuous readjustment of control activities.

Once a careful assessment of the potential and the capacities of existing services has been made, the need for special *in-depth studies* and *research projects* can be established. In-depth studies may be necessary to ascertain the classification of paradigms, to establish local criteria (for case definitions, verbal autopsies), and to investigate outbreaks or operational problems. Special surveys may also complement the monitoring and evaluation procedures integrated into the existing services.

While the position of special surveys does not create a major problem, the position of *research* should be recognized as something that has presented problems in the past and still does so today. There is a need for both operational research and health systems research (HSR), to accompany all control programmes. HSR is emphasized, because *change* is the ultimate goal of HSR. HSR going on as an integral part of a control programme also complements routine monitoring and evaluation in ensuring the itinerative process of the management of control. In particular, it allows the changing patterns of demand and need among the population concerned to be followed. Also, any research or evaluation needs to be undertaken primarily by control staff (staff from existing services, rather than staff not related to control operations, such as university teams). Specialized research teams should try to associate fully with control activities in order to provide the best possible basis for findings to be translated into control activities within a short time-period. This also implies that bi- and multilateral donors should link service support projects or programmes with research/evaluation components.

Community

Contact and communication with the communities as a basis for subsequent involvement and participation have already been stressed as a crucial prerequisite for planning any malaria control. At the strategic level, two major issues should be considered.

The determinants for community involvement are the questions of (1) whether, and how, we know about the demands of the community (an indicator for communication and the understanding of the social and cultural context), and (2) how much decision-making power the community possesses and/or will receive through a control programme.

In addition to these determinants any organizational structure will have to examine how, and how effectively, it will reach the household level. When intervention tools, such as bednets, are used, which are fully household based, the household focus will be crucial for ensuring compliance and assessing impact.

In conclusion, the need is to orient the organization of control rigorously towards *maximizing community effectiveness*: i.e., maintaining efficacy of the tools applied by ensuring an organizational set-up for control that optimizes all steps of the process, from efficacy to community effectiveness. Examples would be the accuracy by which a tool is applied, the compliance of both the users and the providers of the tool, and the coverage to be achieved. Making sure that each step is properly carried out will in turn ensure the effectiveness that provides a major cornerstone for the sustainability of control operations in any setting.

Malaria vaccine research—a game of chess

Kamini N. Mendis

University of Colombo, Sri Lanka

Introduction

Following several decades of research on malaria vaccine development, the field at a glance may present a conflicting picture, with several achievements, and some disappointments and controversies. For example, sporozoite vaccine trials in man with what was thought to be a promising vaccine candidate resulted in a disappointing immune response in vaccinees, raising fundamental questions of whether the immunological effector mechanism in man against sporozoites is mediated by humoral antibodies or whether it is mainly a cellular response, and also some fundamental questions about the immunogenicity of malarial antigens. In the field of asexual vaccine development, on the one hand is a partially successful vaccine trial in humans with a vaccine comprising a synthetic polymer of regions of three asexual blood-stage proteins, two of which whose location in the parasite is still not known; on the other hand are a large number of antigens structurally well defined and characterized, in many of which genes have been cloned but with their candidature being still questionable. Transmission-blocking malaria vaccines present a straightforward, antibody-mediated mechanism, which is potentially promising, but with vaccines facing technical and other developmental issues. These various vaccines are based on the classical approach to vaccination, which is to raise host immunity against the parasite so as to reduce parasite densities or to sterilize an infection.

A newer approach is development of antidisease vaccines which aim to alleviate morbidity by suppressing immunopathology in the host. Antidisease vaccines are based on neutralizing parasite components that induce host pathology, leaving the parasite itself directly unaffected.

Against such a background, I have attempted here to deliver an overview of the state of development of malaria vaccines and present an analysis of the issues that confront the field.

Different antiparasite vaccines against a complex parasite

Several of the different immunological fronts presented by the malaria parasite during its life cycle have been identified as potential targets for antiparasite vaccines. These are sporozoites, the stage that is introduced into the human host by an infective mosquito, and the intrahepatic developmental stages following soon after, which are perhaps best considered together as pre-erythrocytic stages: a vaccine based on these stages could prevent human infection. Next, the asexual erythrocytic stage parasites which are directly responsible for the pathology of the disease, a vaccine against which could reduce pathology and hence morbidity and mortality even if not completely protective. Finally, the sexual stages, gametes, gametocytes and zygotes (and ookinetes) which transmit the infection from man to mosquito, immunity against which could therefore reduce or abolish transmission of the disease in an endemic population. These effects would accrue when each type of vaccine is considered by itself; however, synergistic effects may be expected when they are used in combination.

The rationale for vaccines based on any of these stages was that immunization of various hosts with whole parasites of each of these stages has been able to induce protection or total transmission-blocking immunity. Less significant but not to be discounted is the fact that natural malaria infections in humans have been shown to induce immunity against every one of these parasite stages against which vaccines are being developed (Nardin et al., 1979; Cohen et al., 1961; Mendis et al., 1987); an exception to this are those stages that are present only in the mosquito vector with component molecules not presented to the human host, such as exclusively ookinete antigens. The significance of vaccine candidate antigens being targets of natural immunity is that, in endemic areas, boosting of vaccine-induced immunity may be achieved by natural infection; this, however, may not be an essential requirement for the success of a malaria vaccine.

For several very apparent reasons a vaccine today is conceived of as a subunit as opposed to whole parasite vaccines, either in the form of a recombinant product or as synthetic peptide constructs. Genes coding for several antigens of *Plasmodium falciparum* and some of *P. vivax* have been cloned and sequenced, revealing a feature which seems to be common to many *Plasmodium* antigens; this is that they contain tandem repeats of oligopeptide sequences which often code for immunodominant epitopes (Kemp and Cowman, 1990).

A growing list of 'potential vaccine candidates'

With sporozoite vaccines, a single antigen on the sporozoite surface — the circumsporozite (CS) protein — has been the main focus of studies for a long time. Immunization and even challenge studies have been done in human volunteers, with recombinant and peptide antigens of the *P. falciparum* CS, based on an immunodominant B-cell epitope coded for by tandem repeats of four amino acids (NANP); satisfactory levels of protection were not obtained in these trials. With a trimeric synthetic peptide $(NANP)_3$ conjugated with tetanus toxoid, one of three best responders who were challenged proved to be fully protected (Herrington et al., 1987). In a trial with the recombinant peptide one of six challenged volunteers was protected (Ballou *et al.*, 1987). As for other pre-erythrocytic stage antigens, several liver stage-specific antigens and some shared between liver stages and sporozoites have been cloned in the recent past (Druilhe and Marchand, 1989) but their functional significance remains to be determined. One such antigen, the sporozoite surface protein 2 (SSP2) of a rodent malaria parasite, when used in combination with the CS to immunize mice, protected these animals against a challenge infection (Khusmith *et al.*, 1991).

In the field of asexual blood stage vaccine development not one, but several, potential candidate antigens of this stage are being considered (Anders and Brown, 1990; Kemp and Cowman, 1990; David *et al.*, 1990). Some of the favoured candidates in *P. falciparum* and their present candidature status are mentioned briefly below.

The schizont surface glycoprotein, referred to by various names (PMMSA, P190, gp195, P185, PSA, MSP-1 and MSA-1), chosen because of its merozoite surface location, still retains its candidature for a vaccine because immunization of animals with this antigen has given fairly consistent protection in several trials (Holder, 1988). Monkeys immunized with the native protein purified from *P. falciparum* and also with an NH_2-terminal synthetic peptide of this antigen induced some protection against homologous challenge. Another synthetic peptide derived from the same NH_2-terminal region was used as a component of a multivalent synthetic vaccine in human volunteers in Colombia with encouraging results (Patarroyo *et al.*, 1988). Considerable antigenic diversity exists in this molecule among different strains of *P. falciparum*, and gene sequences from many strains have shown that the molecule contains alternative conserved and variable regions, and that the variable regions are mostly of two types. The equivalent antigen in *P. vivax*, PV200, has been cloned (del Portillo *et al.*, 1991).

The candidature of other antigens is much less clear. MSA-2 is another merozoite surface antigen which holds promise (Anders and Brown, 1990) because of its location, and because monoclonal antibodies against an epitope encoded by sequences within a repeat region of the gene inhibit merozoite invasion *in vitro*. Sequencing of the cloned gene from several strains of *P. falciparum* revealed conserved COOH- and NH_2-terminal sequences flanking strain-variable regions which contain different repetitive sequences.

Then there are rhoptry antigens of merozoites that are discharged onto the red cell surface during the invasion process (Anders and Brown, 1990). Several genes coding for rhoptry protein complexes have been cloned, and these lack the extensive antigenic and structural diversity found in the merozoite surface antigens. Their inclusion in this list is based on successful immunization experiments in a rodent malaria system and because monoclonal antibodies to *P. falciparum* inhibit merozoite invasion *in vitro*. No protection has yet been reported with cloned rhoptry antigens of human malaria parasites.

There is a category of antigens given high priority as they are exposed on the surface of infected erythrocytes. The interest in them stems partly from their association with cytoadherence, a phenomenon which in *P. falciparum* is seen as being linked to cerebral malaria and mortality, and partly because antibodies to surface antigens of *P. falciparum* have been correlated with resistance to infection in an endemic region (Marsh *et al.*, 1989). One of them, PfEMP1, has been characterized by surface labelling and immunoprecipitation (Howard *et al.*, 1988), but the gene has not been cloned.

There are two antigens of unknown location which when isolated from infected erythrocytes partially protected *Aotus* monkeys from *P. falciparum*. A hybrid peptide combining these two plus a peptide from the PMMSA and other sequences in the form of a disulphide-bond linked polymer partially protected human volunteers in the first clinical trial of an asexual blood stage vaccine, performed in Colombia (Patarroyo *et al.*, 1988).

Pf155/RESA is an antigen that is transferred to the erythrocyte membrane after invasion by the merozoite (Perlmann *et al.*, 1984; Anders and Brown, 1990). The gene has been cloned and sequenced and shown to contain two blocks of repetitive sequences which encode immuno-dominant epitopes. These repeats are conserved among different strains and no antigenic diversity has been reported with this antigen. Antibodies against Pf155, both polyclonal and monoclonal, inhibit merozoite invasion *in vitro*, and in a vaccine trial in *Aotus* monkeys fragments of the antigen provided a partial protection against challenge with *P. falciparum* (Collins *et al.*, 1986); this protection was not consistent in subsequent trials. Moreover, the immunodominant epitope of RESA appears to be one of a network of cross-reacting *P. falciparum* antigens and evidence suggests that other antigens and not RESA may well be the target of the effector immune mechanisms.

With sexual stages the picture is more clear, at least as far as potential candidate antigens are concerned. The mechanism is one of antibody-mediated neutralization of mosquito midgut stages which takes effect within a very short period of time. Antigens recognized as targets for transmission-blocking immunity are located on the surface of extracellular gametes, zygotes or ookinetes. Several such antigens, a 230-kDa and 48/45-kDa doublet on gametes and a 25-kDa molecule on zygotes of *P. falciparum* (Carter *et al.*, 1988) and several on gametes of *P. vivax* (Premawansa *et al.*, 1990) have been identified. Two of these, the Pfs25 in *P. falciparum* and GAM-1 in *P. vivax* (unpublished results), have been cloned. Vaccination experiments in a rodent malaria system with a parasite-purified equivalent of the 45-kDa gamete antigen of *P. falciparum* conferred very effective transmission-blocking immunity. What appears to be a consistent feature of sexual stage antigens is that the epitopes involved in transmission-blocking immune reactions are tertiary structure- or conformation-dependent, a feature which delayed the cloning of these antigens because conformational structure is generally not expressed in bacterial systems which were widely used for the construction of DNA libraries. Not withstanding these difficulties, the ookinete antigen of *P. falciparum*, Pfs25, has been cloned (Kaslow *et al.*, 1988). Mice have been successfully immunized with Pfs25 as a recombinant vaccinia vaccine to produce transmission-blocking antibodies (Kaslow *et al.*, 1991).

Extensive as it may seem, the antigenic profile of *Plasmodium* thus far recognized and exploited for vaccines is unlikely to represent all of the potential candidates. For example, evidence is still forthcoming that non-CS antigens may constitute a significant part of the sporozoite surface (Hollingdale *et al.*, 1990; Druilhe and Marchand, 1989; Khusmith *et al.*, 1991). Newer antigens are still being demonstrated as potential targets for immunity against asexual blood stages and sexual stages of *P. falciparum* and *P. vivax*. Antigen selection for malaria vaccines is addressed as an issue separately below.

In summary, in the case of sporozoite vaccines the results of human vaccine trials with subunit vaccines have raised fundamental questions about the immune response to malarial antigens. With asexual blood stage vaccines, although potential candidates among characterized antigens are being explored and some even used in human trials, there is still uncertainty about the degree of protection they can afford in a human malaria vaccine. In the case of transmission-blocking vaccines, we have a fairly good idea what the targets of immunity are but have now to develop vaccine constructs to contain these. We are thus faced with several interesting and important issues in trying to achieve the desired protection with a subunit malaria vaccine, well illustrated in the saga of the sporozoite vaccine.

The hepatic stage may be at least as important a target as the sporozoite for immunity against pre-erythrocytic stages

The development of a sporozoite vaccine was based on raising high-titre antibodies to a very immunodominant and repetitive epitope on the CS protein located on the surface of sporozoites. In the aftermath of the recent failures in human vaccine trials (failure meaning that only one of the best antibody responders was protected when challenged), the results of a spate of studies performed recently have suggested that cytotoxicity against yet another epitope of this antigen rather than antibodies against the repeat region encoding the immunodominant B-epitope may be an important mechanism of protection against a sporozoite challenge (Kumar *et al.*, 1988; Romero *et al.*, 1989; Hoffman *et al.*, 1989; Weiss *et al.*, 1988). Evidence also suggests that infection of hepatic cells may be essential for the induction of immunity against pre-erythrocytic stages (Mellouk *et al.*, 1990). Therefore, contrary to previously held views, recent developments point to the possibility of exploiting immunity against epitopes expressed elsewhere in the CS protein, possibly on the surface of the infected hepatocyte, in a vaccine.

Antigenic polymorphism: is it a pitfall?

Cytotoxic T-cell epitopes on the CS antigen have been mapped to a region of the antigen well outside the repeat region (Dontfraid et al., 1988). It appears that there is only a very limited number of cytotoxic T-cell epitopes in this antigen. In addition, the region in which the cytotoxic T-cell epitope lies is also the polymorphic region of the gene (Good et al., 1988a; Guttinger et al., 1988; Lockyer et al., 1989). Polymorphism of malarial antigens among natural parasite populations is extensive and has been described for both B and T epitopes of many antigens of all stages of the parasite. Among these polymorphic antigens are several that are considered as potential vaccine candidates (Mendis et al., 1991). These include the B epitope of the CS antigen of P. vivax, the schizont and merozoite surface antigens P. falciparum and P. vivax, MSA1 and PV200 respectively, another merozoite surface antigen of P. falciparum, MSA2, erythrocyte surface antigens of both species, and sexual stage antigens of P. vivax and to a lesser extent of P. falciparum. Experimentally, polymorphism of an antigen can indeed influence the immune response to it (De Groot et al., 1989; Guttinger et al., 1988). In the light of existing evidence antigenic polymorphism appears to be one of the important mechanisms of immune evasion by the parasite (Mendis et al., 1991). However, the extent to which this would affect the efficiency of a vaccine would depend on the degree of variability in natural isolates of the targets and/or inducers of immunity. It seems likely that in natural parasite populations the repertoire of variants of a given antigen is finite because the sera of residents of endemic areas who with advancing age acquire a partially protective immunity recognize a wide range of variants (Mendis et al., 1991). It is conceivable that such a situation could be met with a multivalent vaccine construct. However, there is evidence from an experimental situation that even an apparently invariant malarial antigen could undergo variation under vaccine-induced immune pressure (David et al., 1985; Klotz et al., 1987), which suggests that antigenic polymorphism or variation would have to be important considerations in any antiparasite malaria vaccine. There is also the hope that some parasite molecules such as those that are critical for biological function may be conserved, so that these could be deployed for vaccines, but again, as discussed below, most biologically critical functions seem to depend not on one, but on several different mechanisms and pathways (Dolan et al., 1990).

The host is also polymorphic, and so is its immune response

Another subject that has come under close scrutiny since human trials were performed with subunit sporozoite vaccines is the variability of the human immune response to malarial antigens. The T-cell responses to peptides representing the CS antigen of P. falciparum among individuals exposed to intense malaria transmission were found to be highly variable (Good *et al.*, 1988b). Even human immune responses to the gamete surface antigens were found to be very variable among individuals (Carter *et al.*, 1989); this could not be owing to a variable exposure to these antigens because all individuals responded to internal gamete antigens which are not targets of antiparasite immunity. So, it appears that the human immune response to malarial proteins that are sensitive targets of immunity such as the CS and gamete surface antigens are very variable. The reasons for this are probably complex but nevertheless are likely to include: (1) Ir gene (MHC) constraint of immune responses to individual T-cell epitopes; (2) limited number of recognizable T-cell epitopes on these proteins; and (3) T-cell epitope variation among parasites. Many other factors especially in a population being immunologically assailed to the extent of one exposed to malaria and many other parasitic diseases in the tropics probably complicate the outcome of the immune responses to these and other malarial antigens. The constrained recognition of some malarial antigens by humans would cause problems not only for inducing immunity to a malaria subunit vaccine based on such antigens but also for its boosting by genetically different parasite inoculations (Mendis *et al.*, 1990a).

The variability of human immune responses to malarial antigens may also be a consequence of the altered immunological reactivity of endemic populations. There is substantial evidence now that suggests that prolonged exposure to endemic malaria lowers the immune responsiveness of populations, and that this may even be specifically to malarial antigens (Riley *et al.*, 1989; Goonewardene *et al.*, 1990). Recent studies have led to the demonstration of cell populations that may suppress immune responses (Riley *et al.*, 1989; Mshaba *et al.*, 1990). An understanding of underlying mechanisms could lead to improved vaccine constructs.

The immune response can favour the host or the parasite

Studies on the immune response to natural malaria infections have so far focused almost exclusively on the specificity of a response. Other possibly important aspects of the quality of an immune response such as the isotype, avidity and affinity of antibodies need to be explored as they may provide vital clues to important effector mechanisms (Groux *et al.*, 1990).

Immunopathology is a well-recognized entity in malaria and has been considered classically as a possible vaccine-associated hazard. The deployment of subunit vaccines may minimize but not eliminate such risks. Another consideration is that antibodies against the parasite such as antisporozoite (Nudelman *et al.*, 1989) and antisexual stage antibodies (Peiris *et al.*, 1988) have been shown at low concentrations to have the opposite effect on the parasite and enhance parasite development. None of these, it is hoped, may pose serious deterrents to vaccine development at this stage but are worthy of inclusion in a list of considerations.

The right vaccine, the right presentation

Expression and delivery of antigens are presently somewhat central issues, particularly with malaria vaccines which have reached a more advanced state of development such as the CS vaccines and transmission-blocking vaccines based on the Pfs25 antigen. The target epitopes for transmission-blocking immunity appear to depend on the tertiary conformational structure of these molecules (Carter *et al.*, 1988; Premawansa *et al.*, 1990). It appears now that eukaryotic expression is probably essential for correct folding and epitope presentation and perhaps even glycosylation. Yeast and baculovirus expression and the use of mammalian CHO cells are planned.

Delivery systems are bound to be critical for a malaria vaccine. Live vectors have potential particularly for antigens such as the CS protein with cytotoxic epitopes. There is a wide range from vectors such as the pox viruses to bacterial vectors such as *Escherichia coli* or *Salmonella typhimurium* which can be genetically manipulated to express foreign proteins (WHO Meeting, 1990). BCG is a potentially important one in this respect. One malarial antigen, namely the CS protein of a murine malaria, has been used successfully to transform an attenuated strain of *Salmonella typhimurium* for use as an oral vaccine which protected mice from challenge. A successful CS recombinant vaccinia vaccine has also been reported in mice (Sadoff *et al.*, 1988; Aggarwal *et al.*, 1990) and so has a transmission-blocking recombinant vaccinia vaccine of Pfs25 in mice (Kaslow *et al.*, 1991). Malaria vaccines that aim to induce high levels of neutralizing antibodies will incorporate better carrier proteins, more potent adjuvants and may have to use alternative delivery systems such as liposomes and proteosomes.

From monkey to man

Doubts about the validity of criteria for antigen selection, particularly in the case of asexual stage antigens, means that there is a great deal of uncertainty as to when one should proceed to simian and human trials. Animal trials, in this case non-human primate trials, are severely limited by the low availability of non-human primates. Performing vaccine trials with each of the many different candidate antigens may not be feasible. Non-human primates constitute a valuable resource for confirming the candidature status of antigens; however, the question often arises whether a successful simian trial is needed to proceed to human trials and, if not, whether it is necessary to perform trials in monkeys at all? This type of debate is largely spawned by the limited resources available for empirical studies (WHO, 1988).

In the light of issues discussed above, the idea of potential malaria vaccines that would induce partial protection in man but not necessarily a complete sterilizing immunity should be entertained. Here we confront an important issue of vaccine evaluation. Ethical standards which make it imperative to treat *P. falciparum* infections at the lowest detectable levels in the circulation necessarily exclude the selection of vaccines which induce partial protection. An example is presented in the first human phase II asexual blood stage vaccine trial performed in Colombia in which a parasitaemia of 0.5% was defined as the level for termination of a challenge infection by drug cure (Patarroyo *et al.*, 1988). Had this level been lower, the protective nature of the vaccine tested may not have been apparent because in at least two of the five subjects who eventually controlled their infection the parasitaemia rose to nearly a 0.5%. Guidelines for evaluating malaria vaccines which could significantly reduce morbidity and mortality without achieving a sterilizing immunity may have to be reformulated.

A lack of knowledge on some critical aspects of malaria transmission, i.e. the quantitative relationship between the size and frequency of the sporozoite inoculum and disease, has been a major conceptual constraint to vaccine development. For example, could partial protection against sporozoites alleviate the morbidity and mortality in children in hyperendemic regions, which accounts for 25% of childhood deaths in these areas (Greenwood *et al.*, 1987), or would it not affect the malaria picture at all? These are questions to which we would need to know answers before any type of malaria vaccine now being considered can be eliminated from a priority list. There is no indication at all that one of them is potentially for any reason more hopeful than the others.

Have we doubts?

Recent human trials with a CS antigen subunit vaccine led to studies that brought a wealth of information to the field and some changes in concept. It may then be timely to re-examine some of the assumptions underlying the methodology of subunit vaccine development and evaluation. First would be the question of whether subunit vaccines against malaria are even feasible. An effective protection of an animal host against malaria has been achieved by the passive transfer of a T-cell clone (Brake *et al.*, 1988) and experimental evidence of this nature is a reminder that it may indeed be possible to simulate the success achieved by immunizing with a single native antigen of *Plasmodium*, with a subunit vaccine construct.

To vaccinate against malaria, however, is to intervene in a host–parasite system of evolutionary success, and has connotations which cannot be ignored. One is that the natural history of human malaria and immune responses must provide the most important clues for vaccine strategy. It demonstrates too the fallacy of extrapolating information from artificial host–parasite systems to human malaria. Parasite behaviour and immune dynamics in natural host–parasite systems which have evolved together are likely to be different from those of, for example, human malaria parasites newly introduced into a susceptible host.

Secondly, the very fact that the natural immune response to the parasite is poor may indicate that potentially lethal parasite targets are rendered inaccessible to the immune system of the host. If so, the basis of using immunoscreening as a method of selecting potential vaccine candidates might have led to the exclusion of important targets. Should not the parasite genome then be explored either systematically or with a new set of criteria for expressed parasite components other than those readily recognized by the immune system? Relatively few attempts have been made to investigate the functional relevance of parasite molecules with a view to using them as potential immunological targets (Braun-Breton et al., 1988; Adams et al., 1990). Even these attempts may have been thwarted somewhat prematurely by a failure to recognize what seems to be a fundamental feature of biological systems, which is that not one, but multiple mechanisms and diverse pathways underlie all biologically critical functions (Dolan et al., 1990).

Infection without disease?

Thirdly, measures that sustain a selection pressure on the parasite may inevitably be countered by highly evolved parasite mechanisms. From this point of view, antidisease vaccines present a different approach, to alleviate disease without imposing a lethal pressure on the parasite (Clark, 1987; Playfair et al., 1990). Much progress is being made in defining immunopathological pathways and identifying parasite molecules that induce host cytokines and other disease mediators (Taverne et al., 1990; Mendis et al., 1990b). These antigens may not be critical for parasite survival, and may thus have a major advantage of not having to face counter-effects of immune evasion by the parasite. Such antigens will undoubtedly face technical and development issues confronted by other forms of malaria vaccines. However, antidisease vaccines could be expected to reduce childhood mortality effectively in endemic regions and extend life until antiparasite immunity develops at a later age.

Issues facing the development of a malaria vaccine are complex. It is not clear how far we may yet be from achieving this goal. The work of the past decades has laid an extensive foundation of relevant knowledge and technologies, and the goal itself remains as important as ever. Will funding agencies as well as scientists remain committed to this objective?

Acknowledgements

I wish to acknowledge Richard Carter, Peter H. David, Odile Mercereau-Puijalon and Pierre Druilhe for useful discussion.

References

Adams JH, Hudson DE, Torii M, Ward GE, Wellems TE, Aikawa M and Miller LH (1990). The Duffy receptor family of *Plasmodium knowlesi* is located within the micronemes of invasive malaria merozoites. *Cell, 63*, 141

Aggarwal A, Kumar S, Jaffe R, Hone D, Gross M and Sadoff J (1990) Oral salmonella: malaria circumsporozoite recombinants induce specific CD8 cytotoxic T cells. *Journal of Experimental Medicine, 172*, 1083

Anders RF and Brown GV (1990) Vaccines against asexual blood stages of *P falciparum*. In Ishizaka K, Kallos P, Lachmann P and Waksman BH (eds) *Progress in Allergy 41*. Karger, Basel, pp. 491–512

Ballou WR, Rothbard J, Wirtz RA, Gordon DM, Williams JS, Gore RW, Schneider I, Hollingdale MR, Beaudoin RL, Maloy WL, Miller LH and Hockmeyer WT (1987) Immunogenicity of synthetic peptides of *Plasmodium falciparum*. *Science (USA), 228*, 996

Brake DA, Burns JM Jr, Weidanz WP, Vaidya AB and Long CA (1988) Adoptive protection in nude mice against a murine malarial parasite using a cloned T-cell line. *Vaccines, 88*, 85–88

Braun Breton C, Rosenberry T and Pereira da Silva L (1988) Induction of the proteolytic activity of a membrane protein in *Plasmodium falciparum* blood schizonts and merozoites by phophatidyl inositol specific phospholipase C. *Nature (Lond.), 332*, 457

Carter R, Kumar N, Quakyi I, Good M, Mendis K, Graves P and Miller L (1988) Immunity to sexual stages of malaria parasites. In Ishizaka K, Kallos P, Lachmann P and Waksman BH (eds) *Progress in Allergy 41*. Karger, Basel, pp. 193–214

Carter R, Graves PM, Quakyi IA and Good MF (1989) Restricted or absent immune responses in human populations to *Plasmodium falciparum* gamete antigens that are targets of malaria transmission-blocking antibodies. *Journal of Experimental Medicine, 169*, 135

Clark IA (1987) Cell mediated immunity in protection and pathology of malaria. *Parasitology Today, 3*, 300

Cohen S, McGregor IA and Carrington S (1961) Gamma-globulin and acquired immunity to malaria. *Nature (Lond.), 192*, 733

Collins WE, Anders RF, Pappaioanou M *et al.* (1986) Immunization of *Aotus* monkeys with recombinant proteins of an erythrocyte surface antigen of *Plasmodium falciparum*. *Nature (Lond.) 323*, 259

David PH, Hudson DE, Hadley TJ, Klotz KW and Miller LH (1985) Immunization of monkeys with a 140 kiloDalton merozoite surface protein of *Plasmodium knowlesi* malaria: appearance of alternative forms of this molecule. *Journal of Immunology, 134*, 4146

David PH, Barnwell J and Mendis KN (1990) Vivax malaria: strategies for vaccine development based on the hepatic, asexual erythrocytic and sexual stages. In Ishizaka K, Kallos P, Lachmann P and Waksman BH (eds) *Progress in Allergy 41*. Karger, Basel, pp. 531–544

De Groot AS, Johnson AH, Maloy WL, Quakyi IA, Riley EM, Menon A, Banks SM, Berzofsky JA and Good MF (1989) Human T cell recognition of polymorphic epitopes from malaria circumsporozoite protein. *American Association of Immunologists, 142*, 4000

Del Portillo HA, Longacre S, Khouri E and David PH (1991) Primary structure of the merozoite surface antigen 1 of *Plasmodium vivax* reveals sequences conserved between different *Plasmodium* species. *Proceedings of the National Academy of Sciences USA, 88*, 4030–4034

Dolan SA, Miller LH and Wellems T (1990) Evidence for a switching mechanism in the invasion of erythrocytes by *Plasmodium falciparum*. *Journal of Clinical Investigation*, *86*, 618

Dontfraid F, Cochran MA, Pombo D, Knell JD, Quakyi IA, Kumar S, Houghten RA, Berzofsky JA, Miller LH and Good MF (1988) Human and murine CD4$^+$ T cell epitopes map to the same region of the malaria circumsporozoite protein: limited immunogenicity of sporozoites and circumsporozoite protein. *Molecular and Biochemical Medicine*, *5*, 185

Druilhe P and Marchand C (1989) From sporozoites to liver stages: the saga of the sporozoite vaccine. In McAdam K (ed.) *New Strategies in Parasitology*. Churchill Livingstone, Edinburgh, pp. 39–48

Good MF, Pombo D, Quakyi IA, Riley EM, Houghten RA, Menon A, Alling DW, Berzofsky JA and Miller LH (1988a) Human T-cell recognition of the circumsporozoite protein of *Plasmodium falciparum*: immunodominant T-cell domains map to the polymorphic regions of the molecule. *Proceedings of the National Academy of Sciences USA*, *85*, 1199

Good MF, Miller LH, Kumar S, Quakyi IA, Keister D, Adams JH, Moss B, Berzofsky JA and Carter R (1988b) Limited immunological recognition of critical malaria vaccine candidate antigens. *Science (USA)*, *242*, 574

Goonewardene R, Carter R, Gamage PC, Del Giudice G, David PH, Howie S and Mendis KN (1990) Human T-cell proliferative responses to *Plasmodium vivax* antigens: evidence of immunosuppression following prolonged exposure to endemic malaria. *European Journal of Immunology*, *20*, 1387

Greenwood BM, Bradley AK, Byass P, Jammeli K, Marsh K, Tulloch S, Oldfield FSJ and Hayes R (1987) Mortality and morbidity from malaria among children in a rural area of The Gambia, West Africa. *Transactions of Royal Society of Tropical Medicine and Hygiene*, *81*, 478–486

Groux H, Perraut R, Garraud O, Poingt JP and Gysin J (1990) Functional characterization of the antibody mediated protection against blood stages of *Plasmodium falciparum* in the monkey *Saimiri sciureus*. *European Journal of Immunology*, *20*, 2317

Guttinger M, Caspers P, Takacs B, Trzeciak A, Gillessen D, Pink JR and Sinigaglia F (1988) Human T-cells recognize polymorphic and non-polymorphic regions of the *Plasmodium falciparum* circumsporozoite protein. *EMBO Journal*, *7*, 2555

Herrington DA, Clyde DF, Losonsky G *et al.* (1987) Safety and immunogenecity in man of a synthetic peptide malaria vaccine against *Plasmodium falciparum* sporozoites. *Nature (Lond.)*, *382*, 257

Hoffman S, Isenbarger D, Long GW, Sedegah M, Szarfman A, Waters L, Hollingdale MR, Meide PHVD, Finbloom DS and Ballou WR (1989) Sporozoite vaccine induces genetically restricted T cell elimination of malaria from hepatocytes. *Science (USA)*, *244*, 1078

Holder AH (1988) The precursor to the major merozoite surface antigens: structure and role in immunity. In Ishizaka K, Kallos P, Lachmann P and Waksman BH (eds) *Progress in Allergy 41*. Karger, Basel, pp. 72–97

Hollingdale MR, Aikawa M, Atkinson CT, Ballou WR, Chen G, Li J, Meis JFGM, Sina B, Wright C and Zhu J (1990) Non-CS pre-erythrocytic protective antigens. *Immunology Letters*, *25*, 71–76

Howard RJ, Barnwell JW, Rock EP *et al.* (1988) Two approximately 300 kilodalton *Plasmodium falciparum* proteins at the surface membrane of infected erythrocytes. *Molecular and Biochemical Parasitology*, *27*, 207

Kaslow DC, Quakyi IA, Syin C, Raum MG, Keister DB, Coligan JE, McCutchan TF and Miller LH (1988) A vaccine candidate from the sexual stage of human malaria that contain EGF-like domains. *Nature (Lond.)*, *333*, 74

Kaslow DC, Isaacs SN, Quakyi IA, Gwadz RW, Moss B and Keister DB (1991)

Induction of *Plasmodium falciparum* transmission blocking antibodies by recombinant vaccinia virus. *Science (USA)* (in press)

Kemp D and Cowman DF (1990) Genetic diversity in *Plasmodium falciparum*. *Advances in Parasitology*, 29, 75

Khusmith S, Charoenvit Y, Kumar S, Sedegah M, Beaudoin RL and Hoffman SL (1991) Protection against malaria by vaccination with sporozoite surface protein 2 plus CS protein. *Science (USA)*, 252, 715–718

Klotz FW, Hudson DE, Coon HG and Miller LH (1987) Vaccination induced variation in the 140 kDa merozoite surface antigen of *Plasmodium knowlesi* malaria. *Journal of Experimental Medicine*, 165, 359

Kumar S, Miller LH, Quakyi IA, Keister DB, Houghten RA, Maloy WL, Moss B, Berzofsky JA and Good MF (1988) Cytotoxic T cells specific for the circumsporozoite protein of *Plasmodium falciparum*. *Nature (Lond.)*, 334, 258

Lockyer MJ, March K and Newbold CI (1989) Wild isolates of *Plasmodium falciparum* show extensive polymorphism in T cell epitopes of the circumsporozoite protein. *Molecular and Biochemical Parasitology*, 37, 275

Marsh K, Otoo L, Hayes RJ, Carson DC and Greenwood BM (1989) Antibodies to blood stage antigens of *Plasmodium falciparum* in rural Gambians and their relation to protection against infection. *Transactions of the Royal Society of Tropical Medicine and Hygiene*, 83, 293–303

Mellouk S, Lunel F, Sedegar M, Beaudoin RL and Druilhe P (1990) Protection against malaria induced by irradiated sporozoites. *Lancet*, 335, 721

Mendis KN, Munesinghe YD, De Silva YNY, Keragalla I and Carter R (1987) Malaria transmission-blocking immunity induced by natural infections of *Plasmodium vivax* in humans. *Infection and Immunity*, 55, 369–372

Mendis KN, David PH and Carter R (1990a) Human immune responses against sexual stages of malaria parasites: considerations for malaria vaccines. *International Journal for Parasitology*, 20, 497

Mendis KN, Naotunne T de S, Karunaweera ND, Del Giudice G, Grau GE and Carter R (1990b) Anti-parasite effects of cytokines in malaria. *Immunology Letters*, 25, 217

Mendis KN, David PH and Carter R (1991) Antigenic polymorphism in malaria: is it an important mechanism for immune evasion? *ImmunoParasitology Today* (combined issue of *Immunology Today* and *Parasitology Today*), A34–A37

Mshaba RN, McLean S and Boulandi J (1990) In vitro cell-mediated immune responses to *Plasmodium falciparum* schizont antigens in adults from a malaria endemic area: CD8[+] T lymphocytes inhibit the response of low responder individuals. *International Immunology*, 2, 1121

Nardin EH, Nussenzweig RS, McGregor IA and Bryan JH (1979) Antibodies to sporozoites: the frequent occurrence in individuals living in an area of hyperendemic malaria. *Science (USA)*, 206, 597

Nudelman S, Renia L, Charonvit Y, Yuan L, Miltgen F, Beaudoin RL and Mazier D (1989) Dual action of anti-sporozoite antibodies in vitro. *Journal of Immunology*, 143, 996–1000

Patarroyo ME, Amador R, Clavijo P, Moreno A, Guzman F, Romero P, Tascon R, Franco A, Murillo LA, Ponton G and Trujillo G (1988) A synthetic vaccine protects humans against challenge with asexual blood stage of *Plasmodium falciparum* malaria. *Nature (Lond.)*, 332, 158–161

Peiris JSM, Premawansa S, Ranawaka MBR, Udagama PV, Munesinghe YD, Nanayakkara MV, Gamage CP, Carter R, David PH and Mendis KN (1988) Monoclonal and polyclonal antibodies both block and enhance transmission of human *Plasmodium vivax* malaria. *American Journal of Tropical Medicine and Hygiene*, 39, 26–32

Perlmann H, Berzins K, Wahlgren M *et al.* (1984) Antibodies in malarial sera to parasite antigens in the membrane of erythrocytes infected with early asexual stages of *Plasmodium falciparum. Journal of Experimental Medicine, 159,* 1686

Playfair JHL, Taverne J, Bate CAW and de Souza P (1990) The malaria vaccine: anti-parasite or anti-disease? *Immunology Today, 11,* 25

Premawansa S, Peiris JSM, Perera KLRL, Ariyaratne G, Carter R and Mendis KN (1990) Target antigens of transmission blocking immunity of *Plasmodium vivax* malaria. *Journal of Immunology, 144,* 4376

Riley EM, Ousman J and Whittle HC (1989) CD8$^+$ T-cells inhibit *Plasmodium falciparum* lymphoproliferation and gamma-interferon production in cell preparations from some malaria immune individuals. *Infection and Immunity, 57,* 1281

Romero P, Maryanski JL, Corradin G, Nussenzweig RS, Nussenzweig V and Zavala F (1989) Cloned cytotoxic T cells recognize an epitope in the circumsporozoite protein and protect against malaria. *Nature (Lond.), 341,* 323

Sadoff JC, Ballou WR, Baron LS, Majarian WR, Brey RN, Hockmeyer WT, Young JF, Cryz SJ, Ou J, Lowell GH and Chulay JD (1988) Oral *Salmonella typhimurium* vaccine expressing circumsporozoite protein protects against malaria. *Science (USA), 240,* 336

Taverne J, Bate CAW and Playfair JHL (1990) Malaria exo-antigens induce TNF, are toxic and are blocked by T-independent antibody. *Immunology Letters, 25,* 207

Weiss WR, Sedegah M, Beaudoin RL, Miller LH and Good MF (1988) CD8$^+$ T cells (cytotoxic/suppressors) are required for protection in mice immunized with malaria sporozoites. *Proceedings of the National Academy of Sciences USA, 85,* 573

WHO (1988) Report on a meeting on the use of non-human primates in malaria research. *Bulletin of the World Health Organization, 66,* 719–728

WHO (1990) Potential use of live viral and bacterial vectors for vaccines. *Vaccine, 8,* 425

WORKSHOP REPORT AND RECOMMENDATIONS
RAPPORTEUR: JOHN H.L. PLAYFAIR

There has been an important change of attitude towards the complexities of the malaria life cycle and the wealth of different potentially protective immune mechanisms, in that these are now seen as advantages rather than (as previously) drawbacks. Thus it could be visualized that more than one type of vaccine might eventually be successful, depending on the target population, and that therefore one successful product should not deter science or industry from investigating others. With several clinical and field trials already completed and others on the way, it was felt to be essential to proceed according to sound epidemiological principles and without undue drama, with the local community treated as an equal partner. Trials in non-human primates, though useful in many circumstances, should not be looked on as an obligatory part of the development of every candidate vaccine.

Turning to the various types of vaccine the workshop noted that most pre-erythrocytic antigens were still based on CSP subunits, but that several other sporozoite and liver stage antigens were now in pre-clinical development. Both antibody and non-antibody-mediated mechanisms (e.g. cytotoxic T-cells) are being considered. A great variety of asexual blood stage antigens are available and the first trial suggested that they may be effective. Here there is an urgent need for further field trials. With this type of vaccine, particular attention has to be paid to the standard used to evaluate protection — e.g. when to drug-treat parasitaemic patients. It was felt that transmission-blocking vaccines are likely to be most effective in situations of low and moderate endemicity, though in highly endemic areas they may still be useful when used in conjunction with vector control methods or in preventing the spread of vaccine and drug-resistant variants. Finally, the more recent idea of vaccinating against symptoms rather than the parasite (e.g. by trying to block antigen-induced TNF over-production) was worthy of further study, and the whole question of the role of cytokines and other immune components in pathology needs to be better understood. It seems unlikely that different manifestations of pathology in P. *falciparum* (fever, coma, anaemia, hypoglycaemia, acidosis) can be attributed to one single cause, since they can occur separately, and they should therefore be investigated individually.

It is unfortunately as true today as ten years ago that we do not fully understand the mechanism(s) by which immunity leads to protection against any stage of malaria. One consequence of this is that there is no reliable *in vitro* test that would predict a successful outcome in any vaccine trial. However, data are being accumulated on antibody against increasing numbers of antigens and T-cell responses, measured not only by proliferation but by cytokine secretion in patients with varying levels of immunity, which can only improve understanding. The role of T-cells is under particular scrutiny: IFNγ and IL-4 are often assayed separately in order to distinguish between predominantly 'inflammatory' and predominantly 'helper' T-cell functions, corresponding to the TH1 and TH2 subsets of CD4$^+$ T-cells that have been postulated for the mouse; T epitopes are searched for in protein antigens thought to be protective and they can be inserted when required into complex antigens. The workshop discussed the somewhat unexpected finding that the AIDS epidemic has so far not had any apparent impact on malaria in terms either of parasitaemua or clinical symptoms. The role of T-independent mechanisms deserves further study and here, as elsewhere, it was agreed that laboratory-based research (e.g. in universities) still had a lot to contribute.

In keeping with the generally more optimistic attitude referred to in the opening paragraph, it was concluded that some of the objections that have been raised against the possibility of success with vaccines may be more theoretical than real. For example, the MHC restriction in the response to small peptides can often be overcome by extending them by a few amino acids. Polymorphism at the level of parasitic antigens does remain a difficulty, but should not be assumed to be insurmountable. It is worth recalling that protection against *Streptococcus pneumoniae* is effectively achieved with vaccines containing less than half of the 84 serotypes. Autoimmunity as a result of cross-reaction with self antigens could also be a problem, but no more so than with most other vaccines. Looking ahead, the danger that a degree of success in vaccine trials might lead to a slackening of other control measures needs to be kept in mind.

Design and conduct of field trials of malaria vaccines

Peter G. Smith and Richard J. Hayes

London School of Hygiene and Tropical Medicine, UK

Introduction

The period when we are indeed 'waiting for the vaccine' (or, more correctly, 'vaccines') provides an opportunity to give careful thought to the design of the field studies that will be needed to assess the protective efficacies and side-effects of different vaccines, and to quantify their likely public health impact in a variety of ecological conditions. Experience with other disease control tools suggests that there is likely to be great pressure to get promising-looking interventions from the laboratory, through efficacy and safety trials and into disease control programmes in the shortest possible time. This is, of course, a laudable aim, but there is often a tendency to proceed too quickly and interventions may reach control programmes before their likely impact in those programmes has been assessed satisfactorily. This action sometimes leads to prolonged uncertainty and debate about the value of the intervention, which could have been avoided had the appropriately designed evaluation trials been conducted at an early stage. An example is provided by the widespread introduction of BCG vaccination against tuberculosis at a time when efficacy had been demonstrated only in selected populations, mostly in developed countries. Its value in many parts of Africa, Latin America and Asia is still unclear. Another example would be screening programmes for cervix cancer, which were introduced widely before there was any information from properly designed studies on their impact on mortality from cervix cancer. This led to uncertainty about the value of such screening as a public health measure for more than a decade.

Unfortunately, the period of waiting for malaria vaccines has been rather longer than many had hoped, but this wait has enabled substantial progress to be made on trial design and, in particular, the WHO has produced comprehensive guidelines for the evaluation of both sporozoite and asexual blood stage vaccines against *Plasmodium falciparum* malaria (WHO, 1986, 1989). These documents discuss, in considerable detail, issues arising in the design of field trials and it is to be hoped that a further set of guidelines will be developed to cover the special issues associated with the evaluation of transmission-blocking vaccines.

In this chapter we highlight what seem to us to be some of the key issues in the design and conduct of malaria vaccine trials and focus on some of the as yet unresolved problems.

Stages in the evaluation of a vaccine

Initial studies of the properties of a potential vaccine are likely to be conducted in vitro and/or in animal test systems. Those products that show promise in such testing may then be evaluated in human volunteers, in steadily increasing numbers, while safety and immunogenicity are assessed and attempts are made to determine the optimal dose (and dose intervals for multiple-dose vaccines). Selection of the dose may involve balancing any side-effects of vaccination against the immune response induced. The volunteers included in at least some of these studies should represent, to the greatest extent possible, those in whom the vaccine will eventually be assessed in efficacy trials, though pregnant women and young children are likely to be excluded, at least initially. Once there is evidence of immunogenicity and safety, it may be appropriate to conduct trials involving the artificial challenge of vaccinated individuals with malaria parasites in which protection against parasitaemia or disease due to malaria is assessed in comparison with a 'control' group of unvaccinated individuals who are similarly challenged. Depending on the target group for the vaccine, such studies might be conducted in non-immune and/or semi-immune individuals. If, after this series of studies, there is evidence of immunogenicity and safety, and possibly also limited evidence of efficacy based on artificial challenge studies, the move to the field may begin, to test the vaccine under conditions of natural challenge. It is important to note, however, that if the early human studies have been carried out in a situation that is markedly different from the area proposed for field trials, then the safety and immunogenicity studies should be repeated in individuals more representative of those in the trial area. This would be the case if initial studies were in adults but the trial of the vaccine was to be conducted in children or if the initial studies were in an area not endemic for malaria. Not all vaccines are likely to be tested in studies involving artificial challenge but if such studies are not conducted, initial small-scale investigations should be undertaken under conditions of natural challenge as some adverse effects of a vaccine may only then become apparent.

These early clinical trials of a vaccine are sometimes called phase I and phase II studies (WHO, 1985), though where phase I ends and phase II begins is not always clear.

Having successfully passed through such studies, controlled trials to evaluate protective efficacy and side-effects in 'field' conditions should be undertaken. These kinds of study (called phase III) are the main focus of this chapter, but in the last section we discuss also phase IV studies, which are evaluations conducted after a vaccine has been deployed in a control programme, as it is only at this stage that the actual, rather than potential, public health impact can be evaluated and, indeed, it may be very difficult to evaluate efficacy against the more serious end-points, such as death, in phase III studies.

Nature and purpose of field trials

The major purpose of a field trial of a new malaria vaccine is to produce unambiguous evaluation of the protection conferred against malaria and of any adverse effects of vaccination. Schwartz and Lellouch (1967) have drawn a distinction between 'explanatory' and 'pragmatic' trials. The former are conducted essentially to test a scientific hypothesis without specific regard as to whether or not the intervention under evaluation might be directly applicable in a disease control programme. For example, a vaccine that had to be given monthly might be evaluated in such a trial. This schedule might not be feasible for a routine control programme, but if the vaccine proved efficacious in the trial the investigators would be stimulated to develop a formulation of the vaccine that could be given according to a more convenient schedule. In contrast to explanatory studies, 'pragmatic' studies are designed to evaluate a vaccine in circumstances as close as possible to those in which it might be used in the context of a routine control programme, so that any effects measured in the trial might be generalized to estimate the likely impact on disease if there were widespread introduction of the vaccine. Both kinds of study are likely to be relevant in the context of malaria vaccines. In early field trials, the objective may be to provide clear evidence that the vaccine can protect when given in 'near-optimal' conditions, and trials may therefore be of the 'explanatory' type, but it is to be hoped that 'pragmatic' studies will predominate in later phase III trials.

The efficacy and safety of a vaccine can be assessed satisfactorily only if the experience of those who receive the vaccine is compared with that of those in a similar group of individuals who remain unvaccinated. Trials of this kind are difficult to conduct if there are already vaccines available that are known to have some effect against the disease under study and in these circumstances only comparative efficacy and safety may be assessable. This stage has not yet been reached, however, for malaria vaccines and an unvaccinated comparison group is ethically acceptable.

It is important that great caution is exercised in generalizing from the results of a field trial. A vaccine may have variable efficacy in different populations and in different subgroups of the same population, depending on such factors as immune status, the pattern and intensity of transmission, and differing parasite strains. Replicate trials are essential for a proper understanding of how the efficacy varies in different situations. It must be stressed, however, that such trials should as far as possible be conducted in parallel as, if they are not, it may become increasingly difficult to persuade ethics committees that a further trial is justified, and this may cause confusion at a later date (as has happened, for example, with respect to BCG vaccination against tuberculosis).

Design of field trials

General principles

For an unambiguous evaluation of the effects of a vaccine, a field trial should be *controlled, randomized* and *double-blind*, and should be of *sufficient size* to measure the protective efficacy and the incidence of side-effects with adequate precision. Only in very exceptional circumstances should trials be designed in which these features are not present. We have discussed above the importance of a 'control' (comparison) group of unvaccinated individuals, against which to assess the effects of the vaccine. Individuals differ in their susceptibility and exposure to malaria. Some risk factors we understand and can measure (e.g. use of mosquito-nets), but there are some of which we are ignorant. Thus, the only way to be sure that those in the vaccinated group are comparable in these respects with those in the unvaccinated group is to base the assignment of individuals to groups on a *random* procedure. If this is not done, then interpretation of any results of the trial may be severely compromised as there may be underlying differences in the risk of malaria in the two groups independent of any effects of the vaccination. The importance of randomization must be stressed strongly, as without this element it is likely to prove very difficult to convince the scientific community that the results of a trial are unbiased.

A feature that is sometimes more difficult to organize but which is equally important is that neither those measuring the end-points under study nor the participants in the trial should know who has been vaccinated and who has not. In other words, the study should be *double-blind*. Bias may result if participants know whether or not they are in the vaccinated group. For example, if they know they are unvaccinated they may be more likely to use antimalarial drugs or to attend a clinic when they have a fever, and both of these responses may bias the evaluation of the effects of the vaccine. Similarly, the diagnosis of malaria may be biased if the assessor has knowledge of whether the individual is vaccinated or not. To achieve double-blindness (participant and assessor) it is generally necessary to give those in the unvaccinated group a preparation that cannot readily be distinguished from the vaccine under study, either by its packaging or its appearance. For such purposes, a placebo preparation might be used or some other vaccine might be given which is not expected to have any impact on the end-points under study. Whatever preparation is used, it should be given according to the same dose schedule as the trial vaccine if blindness is to be ensured. The labelling of the preparations also needs to be considered carefully. If the two preparations are simply labelled A and B, blindness may be compromised if there are obvious differences in side-effects between those receiving A and B, or if one or more participants develops severe side-effects necessitating the breaking of the code. The preferred option, if logistically feasible, is to prepare individually numbered vials for all the participants, with a confidential code-list showing which numbers correspond to which preparation. Options intermediate between these two schemes may also be used. These and other aspects of the design and conduct of field trials are discussed in Smith and Morrow (1991).

Choice of trial site

The planning of a trial is greatly facilitated if there is good information already available on aspects critical for the design. These include data on: the nature and size of the potential trial population; the incidence rates of the different measures of malaria that would be the end-points of the trial (e.g. attacks of malaria/year in different age groups, the malaria mortality rate); local usage of antimalarial drugs supplied through the health service or commercial outlets; the seasonal distribution and intensity of malaria; and differences between villages and in different years in malaria rates. Data on the amount of migration into and out of the trial area are also required. If these data are not available it may be necessary to conduct 'baseline' studies (including entomological investigations) in the proposed area prior to the start of a trial.

There should be adequate provision for the diagnosis of the malaria end-points under study, and clinical facilities to handle any adverse effects of vaccination. It would be an advantage if the research group undertaking the trial had practical experience of the design and conduct of large-scale field trials. If not, arrangements may be needed to obtain epidemiological and statistical input at an early stage of protocol preparation.

The study population

The choice of the target population for a malaria vaccine will depend on the epidemiological circumstances. In some areas non-immune migrants to a malaria-endemic area may be those at greatest risk from the disease and it would be appropriate to vaccinate persons of all ages. There may be special risks associated with the vaccination of pregnant women and young children and it is likely they will be excluded from initial field trials. Establishing pregnancy by questioning is unreliable, and by urine testing is cumbersome, so it may be advisable to exclude from a trial all women of child-bearing age. Pregnant women and young children are at special risk of malaria, however, and once the efficacy of a vaccine has been established in other groups, special trials are likely to be needed in these groups, with careful monitoring for adverse effects.

In areas where malaria is highly endemic, the burden of malaria is suffered mostly by young children and they would be the target group for a vaccine. In such areas studies of safety might be conducted initially in older persons, but these individuals may provide information of very limited value for assessing immunogenicity and efficacy against malaria end-points.

In general, all individuals in the target group in the communities selected for the trial should be eligible for inclusion, excluding only those who may be especially susceptible to adverse effects, or who may suffer apparent adverse effects independently of vaccination (such as very sick children). Such exclusions should be kept to a minimum if the results of the trial are to have applicability in the context of a routine disease control programme.

A vaccine may both protect the individual and, if given to enough individuals, have an effect on transmission of malaria in the community. Trials to assess effects on transmission are discussed under 'Unit of randomization', below. Note, however, that if the primary objective of a trial is to assess individual protection it may be advisable to vaccinate substantially less than half of those in the target group to ensure that effects on transmission do not decrease the occurrence of malaria in those in the unvaccinated group, as this decrease would reduce the power of the study to detect an effect of a given magnitude.

Nature of the intervention

A vaccine that is to be evaluated in a field trial should be a well-defined product that is reproducible and which shows little batch-to-batch variation. If this is not the case, generalization from the results of a trial may be impossible. The schedule of administration should also be well defined in the trial protocol, with respect to dosage, route of administration and intervals between repeat doses if revaccination is required.

An important consideration regarding vaccines that may have to be administered several times is that applicability in a control programme may be much enhanced if the schedule of vaccination fits in with the timing of other vaccines given in the expanded programme of immunization. If this coordination is done it will be important to assess whether administration at the same time as other antigens impairs the efficacy of either the malaria vaccine or the other vaccines. For this reason, and because of possible adverse effects of vaccination in very young children, it may be decided to address this question only when efficacy and safety have been established in older age-groups.

Since the immune response to the vaccine may be compromised by intercurrent malarial infection, a decision is also needed as to whether treatment should be given to clear parasitaemia, either before or at the time of vaccination. Prior testing for malaria infection, and treatment only of infected individuals, might be possible in the context of a trial, but is unlikely to be a realistic option in a routine vaccination programme. Phase II studies or early phase III trials omitting prior treatment could give valuable information on any effect of intercurrent infection on efficacy. If such an effect is demonstrated, a policy of treating all vaccinees at the time of vaccination could be considered for use in later 'pragmatic' trials.

Unit of randomization

Depending on the objectives of the trial, the basic unit of randomization may be either the individual or the community. In the latter case, whole communities are randomized, so that, within each community, either all of those in the target group are offered the vaccination, or none of them are.

The primary objective of malaria vaccines, other than transmission-blocking vaccines, is to protect the individual, and in early phase III trials of such vaccines the assessment of individual protection is likely to be the main aim. In this case, the individual is the preferred unit of randomization, for three main reasons. First, this design allows the effect of the vaccine on the vaccinated individual to be disentangled from any effect on transmission. Secondly, it is easier to preserve the blindness of the study if individuals within the same community are randomized to receive the active or control vaccine. Thirdly, individual randomization provides greater power, since it avoids the additional variability caused by differences in malaria indices between communities. Figure 1 illustrates the increase in sample size needed if community randomization is used. In this example, it is assumed that 10% of individuals are expected to develop

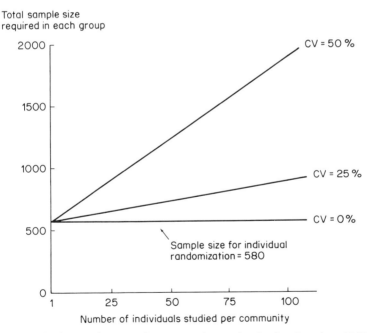

Figure 1 Sample size requirements for community randomization, based on 90% power being required to detect vaccine efficacy of 50%. Incidence of malaria in placebo group is assumed to average 10%, and the between-community coefficient of variation (CV) is assumed equal in placebo and vaccine groups

malaria in the control group, that the vaccine efficacy is 50%, and that 90% power is required. If individual randomization is used, about 580 individuals will be needed in each group. The increase in sample size with community randomization depends both on the number of individuals studied in each community, and on the extent of between-community variation in the risk of malaria, as measured by the coefficient of variation (ratio of mean to the standard deviation, which, for the example, is assumed equal in the vaccine and placebo groups). For example, if the coefficient of variation is 25%, the community-specific risk of malaria in the absence of vaccination is assumed to average 10% and to vary between approximately 5% and 15%; while in the vaccinated group the risk is assumed to average 5% and to vary between approximately 2.5% and 7.5%. It is clear from Figure 1 that the loss of power from community randomization may be appreciable, particularly if there is substantial between-community variation in malaria rates, and if a large number of individuals are studied in each community.

Even if the primary objective is to measure the effect of the vaccine in protecting the individual, it may be decided to randomize by households or compounds rather than by individuals. It may be logistically easier, for example, to give all those in a household the same vaccine, especially if multiple doses of the vaccine have to be given.

Vaccines which provide individual protection may give additional benefit if they offer sufficiently good protection, and can be distributed to a large enough proportion of the population, to have an impact on the transmission of malaria parasites in the community. For this reason, later phase III and phase IV studies might seek to assess the net effect on malaria incidence of vaccinating whole communities, or at least all those in the target groups. For sexual blood stage vaccines, the primary interest is in the effect of the vaccine on transmission. In such cases, the unit of randomization must be the community rather than the individual. The communities should ideally be defined as 'transmission zones' for malaria, covering the effective movements of individuals in a population and those of the mosquitoes to which they are exposed so that, to the greatest extent possible, the problem of infections imported into the community from other communities is minimized. In many areas it may be difficult to define such zones satisfactorily, and in these the effect on transmission that is measured in a trial may be less than that which might be achieved when the vaccine is introduced into the control programme and widespread coverage is attained. It is important to emphasize that the computation of the appropriate sample size must take into account the degree of between-community variation, as illustrated above. Malaria rates often vary greatly between communities over quite small areas, and also show a high degree of variability from year to year within communities. To be able to plan a study of suitable size, it is necessary to have an estimate of this variability and, if it is not available, baseline studies may be necessary before the trial starts.

If communities are the unit of randomization, the absolute minimum number that will be needed to give satisfactory statistical power will be four or five in each group, and often substantially more than this number will be required. Such studies are thus large undertakings. One of the worst kinds of trial design would be to use only two communities: one receiving the vaccine and one not. This is effectively a sample size of one in each group (regardless of the size of each community) and the trial results are likely to be uninterpretable.

Entomological investigations and monitoring are likely to be of special importance in studies aimed at measuring effects of vaccines on transmission.

Trial end-points

A critical aspect in the design of malaria vaccine trials is the choice of the end-points against which to assess the vaccine. In areas where malaria is not endemic, or in non-immune migrants to endemic areas, the definition of malaria may be relatively straightforward: those developing fever and other clinical symptoms of malaria who have malaria parasites in their blood can be classified as cases with little likelihood of error. In places where malaria is highly endemic, however, deciding what is to be called 'malaria' for the purposes of a trial may be more difficult. In these areas, only some of those who are infected may show clinical symptoms, only some with symptoms will progress to severe disease, and only a proportion of these will die. Thus, parasitaemia, mild disease, severe disease, and death from malaria are all possible end-points that may be measured in a trial.

In general, the less common the end-point, the more difficult it will be to conduct trials (as the necessary size of a trial increases according to the rarity of the end-point). Different end-points may be appropriate for vaccines acting against different stages of the parasite life cycle. Thus pre-erythrocytic (and sexual blood stage) vaccines might be expected to prevent parasitaemia, and the incidence of new infections may be the simplest end-point to evaluate. Vaccines against asexual blood stages of the parasite might have less immediate impact in the prevention of parasitaemia but may inhibit parasite levels such that clinical symptoms are less likely to develop, and thus 'clinical malaria' would be the most relevant end-point to assess. To do such assessment, it will be necessary to define 'clinical malaria', and in areas where malaria is highly endemic and many children have fevers for reasons other than malaria, may not be straightforward. To assume that a child who presents with fever and also has parasitaemia is ill because of malaria may be misleading, and may result in overdiagnosis of malaria. This problem may be illustrated with data collected during the rainy season in The Gambia (Greenwood *et al.*, 1987a). Of children who were found to be 'febrile' (defined as a temperature of $> 37.5°C$) during home visits, 59% had malaria parasitaemia. However, 31% of asymptomatic children, examined at the same time of the year, also had malaria parasitaemia. This finding suggests that many of those with fever and parasitaemia had fevers due to causes other than malaria, so that this definition of clinical malaria lacks specificity. The consequence of this definition will be to bias estimates of vaccine efficacy towards zero. The specificity of diagnosis might be improved by restricting the definition of malaria to cases of fever with high levels of parasitaemia, but some individuals will still be wrongly classified as having malaria, as shown in Table 1, and many genuine cases of clinical malaria may be excluded. Given these difficulties, a practical approach is to calculate estimates of vaccine efficacy using two or three alternative definitions of clinical malaria.

One possible solution to the problem of measuring 'clinical malaria' is to include, as well as a vaccinated and an unvaccinated group, a third group of individuals who are given effective antimalarial prophylaxis for the duration of the trial. If malaria parasitaemia can be eliminated from this third group, it is possible to obtain a valid estimate of the efficacy of the vaccine in protecting against malarial fever. This is done by comparing the incidence of 'fever' in the three groups. For example, suppose the average numbers of episodes of fever a year among those in the vaccinated, unvaccinated and prophylaxis groups are 0.7, 1.0 and 0.5, respectively. Thus, malaria is responsible for half of all fevers, as the incidence of fever in those on prophylaxis is 50% of that in the placebo group. An assessment of the efficacy of the vaccine can be obtained by subtracting the 'background' incidence of fevers (that is, the rate in the prophylaxis group) from the rates observed in the other two groups. Thus 'malarial' fevers would be estimated to have rates of 0.2 and 0.5 episodes a year in the vaccinated and unvaccinated groups, respectively, indicating a protective efficacy of 60%.

Whether this strategy would be a practical or an ethical option is debatable. Keeping children on a regimen of effective prophylaxis with 100% compliance over a prolonged period is difficult to achieve, and may interfere with the development of natural immunity. Special measures may be needed to 'wean'

Table 1   Results from a cross-sectional study in The Gambia showing the prevalence and density of malaria parasitaemia according to measured body temperature (Greenwood et al., 1987a)

Temperature (°C)	Malaria parasites in blood film (number/µl)			
	0	<500	500–4999	5000+
<36.5	71%	19%	4%	7%
36.5–36.9	64%	28%	3%	5%
37.0–37.4	70%	28%	2%	—
37.5–37.9	40%	45%	—	15%
38.0–38.4	27%	36%	9%	27%
38.5+	33%	40%	7%	20%

these children off prophylactics at the end of the study. Moreover, to maintain double-blindness, children in the other two groups would have to be given placebo prophylactics according to the same schedule, further complicating the logistics of the trial.

The consequences of malaria infection that are of greatest public health importance are severe disease and death. These are the most important end-points against which an assessment of vaccine efficacy is required, but for both logistic and ethical reasons it may be decided to measure efficacy against parasitaemia or mild clinical malaria, anticipating that these may be used as surrogate measures for the effects that would be seen against the more severe end-points. There are dangers inherent in this approach, however. A vaccine that reduces the proportion of individuals who develop parasitaemia following challenge may not necessarily have the same protective effect against death or severe disease. We have only limited knowledge of why some individuals develop severe disease following infection, while others show few symptoms. It is at least theoretically possible that those who are in the former category may respond in a different way to a malaria vaccine compared with those in the latter category, and thus the efficacy against parasitaemia or mild disease may be markedly different from that against, say, death from malaria. One factor that may be relevant is the strain of the malaria parasite. If infection with some strains is more likely to result in severe malaria, then it is plausible that the efficacy of a vaccine in protecting against the strains resulting in severe malaria may be different from that against the wider spectrum of strains causing mild malaria. It is vital, therefore, that means are found of evaluating impact against the serious end-points also. We believe that this may be done if controlled trials are suitably designed, but there are clearly ethical concerns. We discuss this under 'Ethical issues', below. There are also opportunities to evaluate the impact of a vaccine on mortality as it is introduced into a control programme, in ways such as those outlined below.

It will be important to monitor the development of 'immune responses' in the individuals who are vaccinated. If it can be shown that one or more specific responses are closely correlated with protection against the malarial end-points of interest, then these responses may provide useful surrogate measures of protection in future trials. It is desirable, therefore, that early trials should be designed so that these correlations can be assessed. To do this it will be necessary to take serum samples from all those in the trial both before and after vaccination, and to correlate the change in the immune response with the subsequent occurrence of malaria.

Surveillance for end-points

If parasitaemia and/or clinical episodes of malaria are the main end-points of interest, then surveillance will depend on a combination of cross-sectional surveys to detect parasitaemia and other malariometric indices, and some form of 'continuous' surveillance to detect malarial episodes. To assess the incidence of new episodes of parasitaemia, it may be helpful to treat those who have parasitaemia after the last dose of vaccine, so that all individuals are clear of parasites at the beginning of the follow-up period. When the incidence of parasitaemia is analysed, those who develop malaria and are treated between follow-up surveys have to be added to those who are found to have parasitaemia at the surveys.

The choice of the trial end-points will influence the intensity with which the trial population is monitored following vaccination. If it is desired to detect most clinical episodes of malaria, close monitoring of the participants will be necessary. In areas of high transmission this monitoring may involve visiting each child weekly or more frequently, and enquiring about and measuring the presence of fever, with blood smears being taken from any suspected cases. With this kind of surveillance system it is likely that most cases will be detected (and treated) at an early stage, and there will be relatively few cases of severe disease or death. An alternative to 'active' surveillance of this kind is to adopt a 'passive' system and to rely on cases of malaria reporting to a medical facility for diagnosis and treatment. This policy is likely to result in cases being detected at a later stage in the disease, on average, and may thus enable efficacy to be assessed against end-points of greater public health importance. The extent to which more serious disease is seen will depend both upon how individuals in the population seek treatment for fevers, and upon the accessibility and quality of the medical services. These factors are potentially modifiable in the context of a trial. In general, in those areas where the public health problem of malaria is greatest, the medical services are not well developed, and in the context of a trial it may be necessary to improve them not only to detect cases of malaria arising in the trial, but also to enable any adverse reactions of vaccination to be recognized and treated. Thus, even with a system of passive surveillance, the spectrum of cases detected in a trial may be different, tending to be less severe than those that would occur in the population had the trial not been conducted.

In some circumstances, as discussed in the next section, it may be possible to use death from malaria (or from any cause) as a trial end-point. This policy will usually involve setting up a surveillance system in the (large) trial population to detect all deaths and trying to assign the cause of death by interviewing close relatives about the symptoms and signs preceding death. A verbal post-mortem system of this kind has been used in studies to assess malaria mortality in The Gambia (Greenwood et al., 1987b), and attempts to validate the findings have been encouraging (Alonso et al., 1987). It will be important to monitor mortality from causes other than malaria also as a malaria vaccine may impact on these to the extent that malaria is a contributory factor in deaths due to other causes. The importance of measuring all-cause mortality is illustrated by work by Menon et al. (1990) in The Gambia, who showed that, with the use of a verbal post-mortem procedure, about 25% of deaths in children aged 1-4 years could be attributed to 'malaria', but that fortnightly prophylaxis with Maloprim prevented between 34% and 62% of deaths in this age-range. Similar results have been obtained recently from trials of impregnated bednets (Alonso *et al.*, 1991).

Ethical issues

There are some ethical concerns which are a common feature of all trials of interventions against tropical disease, including trials of malaria vaccines (for example, prior evidence of safety, proper informed consent). There are some special issues, however, that although not unique to malaria vaccines do present important problems in the design of malaria vaccine trials. As discussed above, there is a spectrum of malaria end-points against which a malaria vaccine may be evaluated, ranging from parasitaemia to death, and most public health interest is in the effects on the more serious end-points. There are difficulties in designing trials against these serious end-points, even if malaria is a common cause of death in the population in which a trial is sited. The problems relate to the extent to which it is necessary to make improved provision for malaria case-finding and treatment in the context of a trial. Clearly it would not be ethical to withhold treatment from an individual who was found to have clinical symptoms of malaria but if, for example, the primary effect of an asexual blood stage vaccine is to inhibit parasite proliferation and thus to prevent mild disease progressing to severe life-threatening disease, it will be difficult to observe the effect in a trial in which participants are closely monitored.

We believe that it is important that trials are designed to evaluate the efficacy of a vaccine against the more severe end-points, but it is unlikely that it will be reasonable to do this unless evaluation of the less severe end-points is also undertaken. The timing of these two evaluations may be critical. If a vaccine has been shown to offer protection against the milder forms of malaria, as could be shown, for example, in a relatively small trial with close monitoring of the trial population to detect (and treat) fevers due to malaria, it may then be difficult to convince an ethics committee that a further trial should be performed with mortality as the end-point (which would involve much less close monitoring of the population for episodes of disease). A more acceptable procedure may be to conduct the two evaluations in parallel. Thus, at the same time as defining a trial population that was to be closely monitored for disease due to malaria, a much larger trial population would be defined in which surveillance for severe disease and death would be improved over the existing service but no special attempt would be made to improve the detection and treatment of mild disease. The close monitoring in the smaller trial would probably be required to detect any adverse effects of vaccination, as these would be a potential concern with a newly introduced vaccine. Such monitoring in the larger population would only be for serious side-effects. The relative sizes of the populations in the two trials should be chosen such that the trials would be expected to require the same duration of follow-up so that the answers to both questions (i.e. efficacy against mild and severe disease) would be obtained at the same time.

One objection to the above proposal is that the vaccine would be given to very large numbers of individuals in the mortality trial, before clear evidence of its safety in a field situation was available from the smaller morbidity trial. This problem could be mitigated by phasing the vaccination schedule so that acute side-effects of each dose of the vaccine are evaluated in the smaller trial before the same dose was given in the mortality trial, although this procedure only addresses the problem of immediate adverse effects.

The duration of protection conferred by a vaccine (say, before revaccination is necessary) may be assessed through surrogate measures, such as antibody levels, but should also be measured against clinical disease. For trials in which there is close monitoring of the population, it may be acceptable to maintain a placebo group to establish the variation in protection over time provided that case-finding and treatment of malaria is sufficiently intense so as to prevent serious outcomes in the unvaccinated group. In a population that is not being so monitored, however, it will be necessary to vaccinate those in the placebo group once a protective effect against severe disease has been demonstrated. Assessment of long-term protection may then only be possible through studies conducted after the vaccine has been introduced into disease control programmes, as discussed below.

A further question is whether it is ethical to follow a control group without any intervention, now that data are available showing that selected non-vaccine interventions may have a substantial effect on malarial morbidity and mortality. If it is decided that such an intervention should be provided in the control group, group, then to maintain the validity of the trial it must be given in the vaccinated group also. This policy may have the effect, however, of substantially reducing the incidence of malaria in the study population, so that the power of the trial will be much reduced. Inasmuch as the additional intervention changes the level of transmission of malaria, the results on vaccine efficacy may no longer be applicable to the wider population.

Evaluation when vaccines are introduced into control programmes

The effect of an intervention observed in controlled trials is not always reproduced when the intervention is introduced into routine use in disease control programmes. There may be many reasons (for example, the special nature of populations in which trials were conducted, poorer handling or administration of the vaccine in routine use) and it is highly desirable, therefore, that the efficacy of the intervention in routine use is evaluated. Such evaluations may be valuable also in allowing assessments of the level and duration of protection against severe disease and death, and the efficacy of the vaccine in

differing ecological and epidemiological situations — questions it may be difficult to resolve in phase III trials. We discuss below evaluations that can be
conducted as the vaccine is introduced into a control programme and also
retrospective evaluations that can be done at a later date.

Phased introduction

When a vaccine is first introduced into a control programme, there is a unique
opportunity to plan the introduction in such a way that the public health impact
can be evaluated. Comparison of the incidence of disease before and after the
introduction provides a crude measure of impact, but because of temporal
fluctuations in incidence, independent of the specific intervention, trends may be
difficult to interpret. If the introduction is planned in a phased way such that the
vaccine is not introduced into all places at the same time, it should be possible to
compare the rates of disease in areas with and without the vaccine in use. Phased
introduction of major new interventions is usually the method of choice in any
case, for reasons of logistics and resource constraints. A way in which this
phased introduction might be done is illustrated in Figure 2. Suppose the
country is divided into areas (for example, each area might be that covered by a

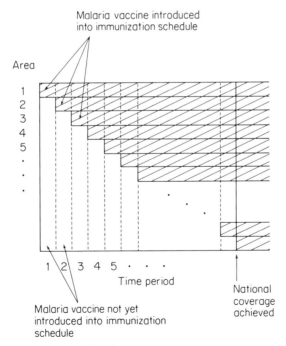

Figure 2   Phased introduction of malaria vaccine into a control programme ('stepped-
wedge' design)

vaccination team or centre). One is chosen *at random* and the vaccine is introduced into the immunization schedule for children in that area. Concurrent with this vaccine introduction a monitoring system is set up to detect deaths from malaria in the area and also in the areas (or a sample of them) where the vaccine is not being given. A second area is chosen, again at random, some time later and the vaccine introduced there, and so on until national (or regional) coverage is achieved. During this time mortality rates are measured in areas where the vaccine has been introduced and in those it has not yet reached. By comparing these rates, a good estimate should be obtained of the impact of the introduction of the vaccine on mortality. Careful allowance has to be made for the asymmetry in the vaccinated and control groups in terms of calendar time.

A design of this form was suggested about ten years ago by Louis Molineaux as a possible means of assessing the impact on mortality of the introduction of antimalarial prophylaxis among children in a malaria-endemic area. A study of this design (called a 'stepped-wedge' design) has been implemented in The Gambia to assess the impact of the introduction of hepatitis B vaccination on mortality rates from liver cancer (The Gambia Hepatitis Study Group, 1987).

Case–control evaluations

When a malaria vaccine has been in use in a control programme for several years, it is important to continue to monitor its efficacy and to assess how any protective effect changes with time since vaccination. As discussed above, it may be impossible to assess long-term protection in a controlled trial because of the difficulty of maintaining an unvaccinated group. In any control programme, however, a proportion of the target population for vaccination miss being vaccinated, and by contrasting their experience, say of death from malaria, with that of vaccinated individuals, assessments may be made of efficacy, and efficacy according to time since vaccination. Of course, such comparisons are more difficult to interpret than results from controlled trials as in a control programme those who escape vaccination, for whatever reason, are not selected randomly and may differ in their exposure or susceptibility to malaria from those vaccinated, independently of any effect of vaccination. Nonetheless, comparison of the malaria rates in the two groups may give a good indication of the effect of vaccination, and adjustments can be made in analyses for known differences in malaria risk factors between the groups. It would be unethical to do such studies prospectively, that is, to follow deliberately a group of individuals knowing them to be unvaccinated without trying to persuade them to be vaccinated, but retrospective evaluation provides an acceptable alternative. In this approach, a surveillance system is used in the population to detect cases of the end-point of interest, say deaths from malaria, and a control group is chosen from persons not dying of malaria similar to the cases with respect to age, sex, place of residence and possibly other known risk factors for malaria. Information is obtained for cases and controls on their history of malaria vaccination, and on other risk factors for malaria, and this infomation may be used to estimate both the protection conferred by vaccination and how this changes with time since vaccination. This 'case-control' method is applicable only if it is possible to obtain reliable vaccination histories from cases and controls but, for example, in many communities mothers preserve carefully the vaccination cards of their children and the relevant information can be extracted from these. A similar case-control approach could also be used with cases of severe malaria, although the choice of controls in this situation may be more difficult. This approach has been used to evaluate the efficacy of BCG, measles vaccine and other standard vaccines in developing countries and is likely to be of value also for the evaluation of malaria vaccines.

Finally, where reliable routine data are available on the incidence of malaria morbidity and mortality, these need to be monitored closely over time, as they may give an early warning of problems with the vaccination programme in particular age groups or geographical areas.

References

Alonso PL, Bowman A, Marsh K and Greenwood BM (1987) The accuracy of the clinical histories given by mothers of seriously ill African children. *Annals of Tropical Paediatrics, 7*, 187-189

Alonso PL, Lindsay SW, Armstrong JRM, Conteh M, Hill AG, David PM, Fegan G, de Francisco A, Hall AJ, Shenton FC, Cham K and Greenwood BM (1991) The effect of insecticide-treated bed-nets on mortality of Gambian children. *Lancet, 337*, 1499-1502

Greenwood BM, Bradley AK, Greenwood AM, Byass P, Jammeh K, Marsh K, Tulloch S, Oldfield FSJ and Hayes R (1987a) Mortality and morbidity from malaria among children in a rural area of The Gambia, West Africa. *Transactions of the Royal Society of Tropical Medicine and Hygiene, 81*, 478-486

Greenwood BM, Greenwood AM, Bradley AK, Tulloch S, Hayes R and Oldfield, FSJ (1987b) Deaths in infancy and early childhood in a well vaccinated, rural, West African population. *Annals of Tropical Paediatrics, 7*, 91-99

Menon A, Snow RW, Byass P, Greenwood BM, Hayes RJ and N'Jie ABH (1990) Sustained protection against mortality and morbidity from malaria in rural Gambian children by chemoprophylaxis given by village health workers. *Transactions of the Royal Society of Tropical Medicine and Hygiene, 84*, 768-772

Schwartz D and Lellouch J (1967) Explanatory and pragmatic attitudes in therapeutic trials. *Journal of Chronic Diseases, 20*, 637-648

Smith PG and Morrow RH (eds) (1991) *A Manual for Field Trials of Interventions against Tropical Diseases*, Oxford University Press, Oxford

The Gambia Hepatitis Study Group (1987) The Gambia hepatitis intervention study. *Cancer Research, 47*, 5782-5787

World Health Organization (1985) Principles of malaria vaccine trials, WHO, Geneva. Document TDR/IMMAL-FIELDMAL/VAC/85.3

World Health Organization (1986) Guidelines for the epidemiological evaluation of *Plasmodium falciparum* sporozoite vaccines, WHO, Geneva. Document TDR/MAP/SVE/PF/86.5

World Health Organization (1989) Guidelines for the evaluation of *Plasmodium falciparum* asexual blood-stage vaccines in populations exposed to natural infection, WHO, Geneva. Document TDR/MAP/PF/89.5

WORKSHOP REPORT AND RECOMMENDATIONS
RAPPORTEUR: LOUIS MOLINEAUX

Field trials of malaria vaccines should answer questions concerning their potential for use for malaria control. There are two main applications of malaria vaccines envisaged.

In the first the objective of vaccination is to prevent infection in human and mosquito, and to reduce/interrupt transmission; the vaccine is likely to include antigens from all parasite life-stages; the intervention strategy is human vaccination combined with vector control; this approach will apply to areas of low to moderate transmission and stability.

In the second approach the objective of vaccination is to modify infection to prevent or alleviate disease; the vaccine will consist of asexual blood stage antigens, with the possible addition of antigens from the sexual stages to prevent the selection of vaccine-resistant parasites; the intervention strategy is to vaccinate early in life, counting on natural boosting for maintenance of immunity. This approach will apply in areas of high transmission and stability.

Field trials, however, will start with simpler questions and the separate evaluation of vaccine components that will eventually be combined. The trials raise both technical and ethical issues; these include study design and impact end-points and their detection.

Technical issues

There are three main basic designs: the double-blind comparison of individuals, the double-blind comparison of communities, and open (i.e. not double-blind) trials, for example in control programmes. Protection by pre-erythrocytic and asexual blood stage vaccines will first be assessed in double-blind comparison between individuals; if protection is achieved, double-blind comparison between communities is unlikely to get ethical approval, and further evaluation will be in open trials. Double-blind comparison between communities is likely to be justified only for sexual stage vaccines, after comparing vaccinated and unvaccinated individuals in terms of infectivity to vectors.

Impact end-points may include: infection, disease, severe disease and death in man and infection in the vector. In humans, the more active the case detection, the more the spectrum of detected malaria shifts towards asymptomatic infection. Figure 1 shows the impact indicators for the different types of field evaluation likely to be used for the three main types of vaccine.

The issues concerning end-points used as indicators of vaccine efficacy are particularly important in the evaluation of impact of asexual blood stage vaccines and specifically on the use of mortality as an end-point. The arguments for including mortality as an end-point in the initial (double-blind) trials are clearly spelled out in the Smith and Hayes chapter.

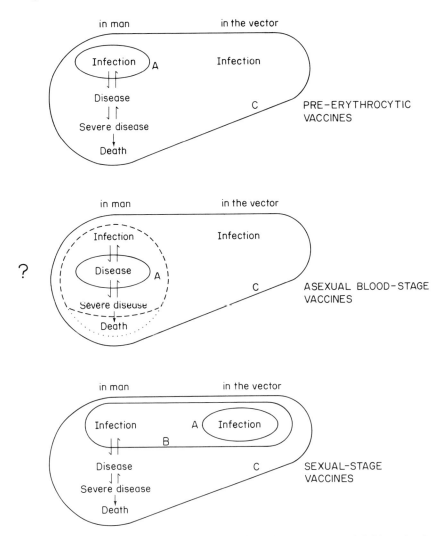

Figure 1 Likely impact indicators by type of vaccine and type of field evaluation (A = double-blind comparison between individuals; B = double-blind comparison between communities; C = evaluation of control programmes)

The following objections were made in the discussion and should be carefully considered:

(1) The widespread and uncontrolled use of antimalarials may maintain a low baseline mortality.

(2) Availability and quality of treatment are likely to be, or should be, improved in trial populations.

(3) For the assessment of safety, it may be imprudent to jump quickly to the large numbers required to measure impact on mortality; if the risk of toxic side-effects is associated with exposure to malaria, it cannot be assessed before the assessment of protection.
(4) The duration of protection should be determined in relatively small numbers before vaccinating large numbers.
(5) Data presented by Brian Greenwood show that chemoprophylaxis reduces malarial disease and malarial deaths by the same percentage; this implies that measurement of disease as an indicator is an acceptable substitute for use of mortality in assessing vaccine efficacy.
(6) The most important desired impact is the long-term prevention of mortality, and early (double-blind) trials will not last long enough to assess this.

Proposals to include chemoprophylaxis in a double-blind evaluation of asexual blood stage vaccines in individuals raise several objections:

(1) It is too complicated logistically.
(2) Chemoprophylaxis has been observed to decrease the frequency of fevers without parasitaemia (if the mechanism is removal of malarial immunosuppression, however, those fevers are still legitimately attributable to malaria).
(3) Populations do find out which is the placebo prophylactic.
(4) Drugs given for prophylaxis may in fact be used for treatment, and this may constitute an ethical objection to placebo prophylaxis.
(5) Chemoprophylaxis may be effective against all species of malaria parasites, and vaccination against one only.
(6) 'Perfect' prophylaxis prevents the acquisition of natural immunity.
(7) Developing drug resistance may invalidate the trial design.

Other technical issues to be considered include:

(1) the use of mathematical modelling to explore vaccination strategies;
(2) the need to detect possible changes in the parasite under immune pressure;
(3) the need to conduct or repeat phase I and phase II trials in the areas selected for field trials.

Ethical issues

(1) Field trials of a particular vaccine should be conducted in populations likely to become targets for vaccination with that vaccine, should it prove effective.
(2) What malaria care should be offered to the study population (vaccinated and controls)? If we advocate the universal promotion of better means of diagnosis and treatment, should we not implement these in populations undergoing field trials?

Recommendations

(1) The problems of how to design field trials of malaria vaccines will become increasingly complicated as there is an increasing number of candidate antigens, and their various combinations could generate a large number of candidate vaccines. At the same time there is pressure to go rather quickly to field testing. There is therefore an urgent need for further development of guidelines on how decisions to undertake field trials are taken, on planning and evaluation of trials, and on how to report results and their implications.

(2) There is also a need for some related basic epidemiological research, such as:

  (a) the epidemiology of malarial disease and death;

  (b) the immunology-epidemiology of malaria, including particularly the transition from passive to active immunity in children born into stable malaria areas, including situations of both seasonal and perennial transmission.

(3) The development of diagnostic and therapeutic services and of malaria information systems is desirable per se and will also be very useful for the selection of areas for vaccine trials and for the planning and evaluation of those trials.

Postscript

Louis H. Miller

National Institute of Allergy and Infectious Diseases, NIH, Bethesda, MD, USA

Malaria remains a problem today because the tools to combat it are inadequate, not simply because we are unable to apply the tools at hand. New technologies could have a major impact on malaria control. DDT was one such technology that spurred the WHO malaria eradication programme and led to the eradication of malaria throughout the Mediterranean basin and near-eradication in India and Sri Lanka. What should we be doing to develop strategies for today and for the future?

Because of the magnitude of the problem of malaria we must use the presently available tools as effectively as possible. These should be evaluated in each country and in separate localities within each country. The dynamic nature of malaria and the multiple variables that determine the problem demand multiple solutions to be tailored to each situation. This will require scientists in each area evaluating the best approach to limit malaria. For this, we need scientists from endemic countries, trained in the varied disciplines related to malaria, to study in their own regions the best control methods. It should be possible to attract the best intellects from endemic countries who are committed to problems of their people and who better understand their customs. These local scientists then can work with the malaria control programmes to develop the best, cost-effective control methods.

From previous experience with DDT and malaria eradication, any tool, no matter how powerful, must be monitored carefully from the initial successes through to the long-term period of control and even after eradication. A percentage of all control money should go to evaluate the effectiveness of the programme on a continual basis and to modify or even abandon methods as they become less effective. How often is this given lip service and not included as an effective arm of every programme? It is common to put a great effort into the evaluation of a new tool (for example, permethrin-impregnated bednets), but once accepted for widespread use the new tool needs continual re-evaluation. This again is best done locally in the context of research within endemic countries.

Because of the magnitude of the problem of malaria, we must convince the funding agencies of the importance of basic research to develop new tools for malaria control and eradication. Funding agencies and administrators often like to define areas of research in terms of near-term and long-term projects. It is impossible, however, to put a time-frame on projects that are exploring basic biological questions and not purely an engineering problem. In 1911 Simon Flexner, Director of the Rockefeller Institute of Medical Research, stated that the discovery of a polio vaccine was only a few years away. In 1949 Macfarlane Burnet, being more cautious than Flexner, placed the time-frame in decades to solve the problem of growing polio in non-neuronal tissue. Yet, in that same year, Enders, Weller and Robbins published their work on the culture of the polio virus that opened the way for the Salk and Sabin vaccines. It is evident that the time-frame for the pay-off from basic research cannot be predicted.

From the early part of the century there has been a conflict between those who felt that all effort should go toward treating the sick and dying with whatever means were at hand and those who saw the need to develop new ways to control malaria. The League of Nations committee on malaria stated in 1925 that, despite the importance of the discovery that anopheline mosquitoes transmit malaria, that knowledge had not had a great impact on disease in the endemic areas. The committee suggested that physicians should stop dipping for larvae and treat patients in the clinics who were dying of malaria. It is curious that treatment of patients (methods for ameliorating the problem immediately) and research should be considered mutually exclusive.

Each of the three areas of research — on the vector, on chemotherapy, and on vaccines — deserve support for their potential for dramatically changing the impact of malaria. Despite what we sometimes read and hear, vaccines are not overfunded. The other areas are underfunded.

Of the anopheline vectors, the *Anopheles gambiae* complex presents unique problems in control. First, wherever *An. gambiae* has been introduced, be it an island in the Indian Ocean, Brazil or Egypt, the result was epidemics of malaria in areas where malaria had previously been relatively easy to control. The problem was only brought under control after *An. gambiae* was eradicated. Second, it dominates an area of the world where childhood mortality is high from malaria. If the vectorial capacity of this species could be reduced, other methods of control might prove more effective. The high vectorial capacity of this species also may play a role in excessive morbidity and mortality in Africa. The extraordinary number of infectious bites transmit many parasite clones, some of which may be virulent in semi-immune children. How to affect this?

There is a new programme at the World Health Organization to modify the vectorial capacity of mosquito vectors. The programme will focus initially on factors in the mosquito that would kill the parasite or block the parasite's development and on methods to introduce the genes for these factors into vector populations. There are two observations that make me optimistic about the feasibility of such an undertaking. First, it has been assumed that the parasite is able to mutate to escape any barrier in the mosquito that we might introduce, as if the possibilities to circumvent barriers are unlimited. This may not be the case.

Mammalian malarias are transmitted by anopheline mosquitoes, although most man-biting anopheline species do not transmit malaria. Culicine mosquitoes do not carry mammalian malaria despite the continual exposure of many of these species to humans and the malaria parasites they carry. This becomes even more difficult to understand when we consider that *P. falciparum* evolved from an avian malaria (Waters and McCutchan, in press) that are transmitted by culicine mosquitoes. There must be some block to the development of the parasite in culicine mosquitoes that is impossible for the parasite to overcome.

Second, there are ways to introduce genes into field populations. For example, the P element first appeared in *Drosophila melanagaster* about 1950 and now is found in most flies of this species around the world. The spread of the P element is non-Mendelian in that it is a transposable element that replicates and moves between the chromosomes in the germ line. Such a transposable element might make the introduction of refractory genes into mosquito populations feasible.

Quite apart from the potential of this new approach, basic research on vector biology should attract a group of young scientists into vector research. Some will be curious about other aspects of vector biology and make a broader contribution than narrowly defined by the goal of modifying the vector.

Chemotherapy is tied to a narrow base of unique agents that include the quinine-related group (chloroquine, mefloquine), antibiotics, a phenanthrene derivative, sulphonamides and antifolates (pyrimethamine and proguanil), and artemesinine derivatives. There is a need to identify biochemical pathways unique to the malaria parasite. One possible area to be explored is haemoglobin digestion. The parasite must reorganize haem into a non-toxic compound, haemozoin pigment. The structure of haemozoin has recently been described (Slater *et al.*, 1991), but it is unknown whether haemozoin pigment is formed by enzymic conversion of haem or is a product of a purely chemical reaction. Whatever, it may be possible to disrupt the formation of haemozoin pigment and thus kill the parasite.

Another approach is to reverse chloroquine resistance. Chloroquine is on the shortlist of drugs that have had a major impact on human health. It will not be easy to replace because of its safety, efficacy and cost. This leaves two problems that are probably quite different and need exploring. First, what is the mechanism of chloroquine action; and, second, what is the mechanism of chloroquine resistance? It should be only a short time before the gene responsible for chloroquine resistance in *P. falciparum* has been identified. The gene has been located on a 200-kb region of chromosome 7 (Wellems *et al.*, 1991). The identification of the gene should open the way for drug design to reverse chloroquine resistance.

Vaccines are probably the most misunderstood area in malaria research. Those in the field and in the funding agencies should stop reading every news release. Unless malaria parasites can be grown outside of the erythrocyte, malaria vaccines will have to be designed as subunit vaccines. The development of subunit vaccines is in its infancy, and only the hepatitis B vaccine has been highly effective, in large part because the membrane protein forms membrane-bound vesicles when expressed in yeast. The subunit approach does, however, offer certain advantages that have not yet been fully explored. For example, the T epitopes of multiple proteins can be incorporated into one recombinant immunogen.

Technical problems facing the field at this time are where recombinant antigens will be made and how to test asexual erythrocytic vaccines. If the antigen, for structural reasons, cannot be made in bacteria, most laboratories cannot handle other expression systems as effectively as industry. Industry has little interest in vaccine development and is in general not interested in absorbing the costs of development. Testing of immunogens requires the availability of monkeys unless a cheaper and more readily available model can be developed. Testing in humans introduces the expense of good manufacturing procedures (GMP), clearing through regulatory agencies and large field studies. This would be limited to the few most promising immunogens. If the chance of finding the best immunogen requires the testing of multiple ones, then the costs are, of necessity, large. The sporozoite vaccine had industrial interest, the support of the US military and other agencies and is still in the early stages of evaluation. Furthermore, the testing of a sporozoite vaccine in humans is far easier than the testing of an asexual vaccine.

The transmission-blocking vaccine may enable the accomplishment of eradication that has eluded us in countries such as India and Sri Lanka, where malaria is still a major problem and a continual drain on the health budget. If insecticides and the WHO malaria eradication programme almost eradicated malaria from Sri Lanka in 1963, then the addition of a transmission-blocking agent to the other modalities of malaria control may accomplish what had previously eluded the eradication programme.

When children are dying from malaria, as in Africa, and the problem is a recurring one as in the Indian subcontinent, it is difficult to accept the slow and unpredictable course of basic research. This attitude, although completely understandable, must be resisted because the field needs the quantum leap in control methods made possible through discoveries. In the case of chloroquine, it took hundreds of years to develop, but none today would argue that the effort wasn't worth it.

References

Slater AFG, Swiggard WJ, Orton BR, Flitter WD, Goldberg DE, Cerami A and Henderson GB (1991) An iron–carboxylate bond links the heme units of malaria pigment. *Proceedings of the National Academy of Sciences of the USA*, 88, 325–329

Waters AP, Higgins DG and McCutchan TP (1991) *Plasmodium falciparum* appears to have risen as a result of lateral transfer between avian and human hosts. *Proceedings of the National Academy of Sciences of the USA*, 88, 3140–3144

Wellems TE, Walker-Jonah A and Panton LJ (1991) Genetic mapping of the chloro-quine-resistance locus on *Plasmodium falciparum* chromosome 7. *Proceedings of the National Academy of Sciences of the USA*, 88, 3382–3386